Practical Guide to Hereditary Breast and Ovarian Cancer II

Akihiro Sakurai • Hideko Yamauchi
Aikou Okamoto
Editors

Practical Guide to Hereditary Breast and Ovarian Cancer II

Annual Meeting of the Japanese Organization of Hereditary Breast and Ovarian Cancer 2022

Springer

Editors
Akihiro Sakurai
Department of Medical Genetics and Genomics
Sapporo Medical University
Sapporo, Hokkaido, Japan

Aikou Okamoto
Department of Obstetrics and Gynecology
The Jikei University School of Medicine
Tokyo, Japan

Hideko Yamauchi
University of Hawaii Cancer Center
Honolulu, HI, USA

ISBN 978-981-96-4328-8 ISBN 978-981-96-4329-5 (eBook)
https://doi.org/10.1007/978-981-96-4329-5

This Springer imprint is published by the registered company Springer Nature Singapore Pte Ltd.
The registered company address is: 152 Beach Road, #21-01/04 Gateway East, Singapore 189721, Singapore

Foreword

This Year Book summarizes the topics presented at the 2nd Annual Meeting of the Japanese Organization of Hereditary Breast and Ovarian Cancer held in 2022. The following are some of the medical and scientific topics related to hereditary breast and ovarian cancer (HBOC) covered in this publication:

The effective use of poly (ADP-ribose) polymerase (PARP) inhibitors for BRCA1/2 mutation-positive patients is extending beyond ovarian and breast cancer to other BRCA-related cancers, highlighting the importance of understanding the mechanisms of their action. As the number of individuals undergoing risk-reducing salpingo-oophorectomy increases, there has also been an increase in cases of occult cancer. How should these cases be managed? What should be the current state of surveillance before and after risk-reducing surgery? Additionally, how can we ensure that the general public understands these issues?

Furthermore, this publication delves into the latest advancements in genetic testing and counseling for individuals at risk of hereditary breast and ovarian cancer. The role of personalized medicine in improving patient outcomes is also included. The importance of multidisciplinary approaches in the management of HBOC, involving geneticists, oncologists, and surgeons, is emphasized to provide comprehensive care.

Each topic is accompanied by the latest insights from leading experts, making this Year Book an invaluable resource for those involved in the management of HBOC, ovarian cancer, breast cancer, and HBOC-related cancers. The information presented here not only aids in clinical practice but also helps in formulating policies for better healthcare delivery.

I would like to express my deep gratitude to Drs. Akihiro Sakurai, Aikou Okamoto, and Hideko Yamauchi for their significant contributions to the editing of this book. Their dedication and expertise have been instrumental in making this publication a comprehensive and authoritative resource.

Tokyo, Japan
November 2024

Daisuke Aoki

Contents

Chapter 1
RRSO and Occult Cancer

Haruhiro Kondo

Abstract Compared to women without BRCA germline pathogenic variants, women with pathogenic variants are at a higher lifelong risk of developing ovarian cancer. There is no conclusive methodology for the early diagnosis of ovarian cancer.

In contrast, hereditary breast and ovarian cancer (HBOC) syndrome is a disease concept that can be diagnosed and allows for subsequent surveillance and risk-reducing surgery. Only risk-reducing salpingo-oophorectomy (RRSO) can reduce the risk of death in ovarian cancer. But after RRSO, risk for a primary peritoneal carcinoma has been reported in some studies, and there have also been reports of occult cancer being discovered through pathological examination after surgery. With the partial approval of diagnostic and therapeutic approaches for HBOC under insurance, the diagnosis rate for these conditions has improved owing to the increased use of genetic counseling and the expanded provision of information. In addition, the need for RRSO has permeated, and currently, several patients are undergoing RRSO. Moreover, it is necessary to educate patients regarding ovarian cancer at the time of breast cancer diagnosis. Laparoscopic RRSO is a procedure that can be conducted safely, but long-term follow-up is needed to monitor the post-operative development of peritoneal cancer and adverse events. Furthermore, a more detailed histopathological diagnosis will allow for the identification of small abnormalities in the fallopian tube. Considering the significance of such lesions, we believe that long-term treatment information and follow-up are of paramount importance.

Keywords RRSO · Occult cancer

H. Kondo (✉)
Department of Obstetrics and Gynecology, St. Marianna University School of Medicine, Kawasaki, Japan
e-mail: haru@marianna-u.ac.jp

A. Sakurai et al. (eds.), *Practical Guide to Hereditary Breast and Ovarian Cancer II*, https://doi.org/10.1007/978-981-96-4329-5_1

Compared to women without BRCA germline pathogenic variants, women with the pathogenic variants are at a higher lifelong risk of developing ovarian cancer. Although the prevalence of ovarian cancer in Japan is 3.1%, the prognosis of advanced ovarian cancer is not favorable. Ovarian cancer is a malignant gynecological disease with a poor prognosis; [1] there is no conclusive methodology for the early diagnosis of ovarian cancer.

In contrast, hereditary breast and ovarian cancer (HBOC) syndrome is a disease concept that can be diagnosed and allows for subsequent surveillance and risk-reducing surgery. According to the NCCN guidelines [2], investigations that combine transvaginal ultrasound and CA125 examination are considered for women between the ages of 30 and 35 years at the discretion of the attending physician; however, the benefits of the method have not been established. Reportedly, only risk-reducing salpingo-oophorectomy (RRSO) can reduce the risk of death in ovarian cancer [3–9] (Table 1.1).

Therefore, ideally, women with BRCA pathogenic variants are recommended to undergo RRSO at the age of 35–40 years, and if these women have family members who developed ovarian cancer at a younger age, the age of onset should be regarded as the ideal age for undergoing RRSO. However, at present, the number of BRCA genetic tests conducted in Japan is considerably lesser than that in other countries, and thus, the percentage of patients with HBOC undergoing RRSO is quite low [10]. However, since April 2020, genetic testing and counseling for patients with breast cancer as well as RRSO for women with BRCA germline pathogenic variants

Table 1.1 *BRCA* pathogenic/likely pathogenic variant-positive management (surgical risk reduction with bilateral salpingo-oophorectomy)

Based on age-related risks of ovarian/fallopian tube cancer:
BRCA1: Recommend RRSO between 35 and 40 years
BRCA2: Because ovarian cancer onset in patients with *BRCA2* P/LP variants is an average of 8–10 years later than in patients with *BRCA1* P/LP variants, [8] it is reasonable to delay RRSO for the management of ovarian cancer risk until age 40–45 years in patients with *BRCA2* P/LP variants unless age at diagnosis in the family warrants earlier age for consideration of prophylactic surgery
CA-125 and pelvic ultrasound are recommended for preoperative planning
See Risk-Reducing Salpingo-Oophorectomy (RRSO) Protocol in NCCN Guidelines for Ovarian Cancer. Appropriate surgical and pathologic expertise is strongly recommended. Sectioning and extensively examining the fimbria (SEE-FIM) protocol for pathologic assessment and pelvic washings should be performed
In addition, in premenopausal individuals, oophorectomy likely reduces the risk of developing breast cancer, but the magnitude is uncertain and may be gene specific
Address bone health, cardiovascular health, psychosocial health, neurologic health, sexual health, and generalized quality-of-life aspects of undergoing RRSO. Consider preoperative menopause management consultation if the patient is still premenopausal at the time of RRSO
Hormone replacement therapy is generally not contraindicated and thus should be discussed with premenopausal patients who do not have a personal history of breast cancer

NCCN Clinical Practice Guidelines in Oncology (Genetic/Familial High-Risk Assessment: Breast, Ovarian, and Pancreatic)

for ovarian cancer prevention have been covered by insurance in Japan. Therefore, the number of RRSO cases is expected to increase.

The risk-reducing effect of RRSO on breast and ovarian cancers was reported in a meta-analysis by Rebbeck et al. [7] in 2009; the authors reported that RRSO reduces the risk of ovarian cancer by 79% and that of breast cancer by 51%. Ovariectomy before menopause is expected to reduce the risk of development of breast cancer, which is an estrogen-dependent tumor; however, since many cases of HBOC are triple-negative cancers, it is speculated that there exist other mechanisms besides hormonal action. Domchek et al. [8] reported in a prospective cohort study of 2482 women with BRCA germline pathogenic variants that RRSO reduced the total mortality by 60%. This was followed by a meta-analysis conducted by Marchetti et al. [11], in which RRSO was reported to reduce the total mortality by 68%. The reduction in overall mortality was similar both before and after menopause, indicating that the increased risk of cardiovascular events owing to premature menopause does not offset the risk reduction of breast and ovarian cancer after RRSO, and the risk of breast cancer from hormone replacement following RRSO did not increase either.

RRSO is intended to reduce the risk of ovarian cancer development, but does not completely eliminate the risk of gynecological cancer development. Cases of peritoneal cancer after RRSO have been reported [12], and instances of peritoneal cancer occurring in 0.5–4.3% of patients who underwent RRSO have also been reported [3–6, 9, 13]. We found that occult cancers and serous tubal intraepithelial carcinoma (STIC), which do not show abnormal findings in various tests conducted before RRSO, can be diagnosed only via detailed postoperative histopathological examination, and various reports indicate that invasive or intraepithelial ovarian cancers, including fallopian tube cancer and peritoneal cancer, have been diagnosed in 2.2%–4.6% of patients [4, 5, 7, 14].

The NCCN guidelines provide a detailed description of the RRSO methodology (Table 1.2).

With regard to the pathological examination of excised specimens, the removed fallopian tube was subjected to the sectioning and extensively examining the fimbriated end (SEE-FIM) protocol proposed by the College of American Pathologists (CAP) in 2006. It was introducing a longitudinal incision into the tubal fimbria and preparing sections at 2–3 mm intervals from the remaining ovaries and fallopian tubes for evaluation [15]. The SEE-FIM protocol can help cut out approximately 60% of the fallopian tube surface, which is important for a more detailed pathological examination [16]. Furthermore, in addition to morphological evaluation, we performed p53 and Ki-67 immunostaining based on the large number of diagnoses of STIC, which is a precancerous condition of high-grade serous adenocarcinoma [17] (Fig. 1.1).

The isthmus and ampulla are cut transversely at 2- to 3-mm intervals [15] (Fig. 1.2).

While RRSO preliminarily reduces the risk of ovarian cancer, conducting a thorough histopathological examination also seems to be effective for the diagnosis of occult cancer and prediction of the subsequent onset of peritoneal cancer. Reportedly,

Table 1.2 Risk-reducing salpingo-oophorectomy (RRSO) protocol

Perform minimally invasive laparoscopic surgery
Survey upper abdomen, bowel surfaces, omentum, appendix (if present), and pelvic organs
Biopsy any abnormal peritoneal findings
Obtain pelvic washing for cytology (50 cc normal saline instilled and aspirated immediately)
Perform total BSO, removing 2 cm of proximal ovarian vasculature/IP ligament, all tube up to the cornua, and all peritoneum surrounding the ovaries and tubes, especially peritoneum underlying areas of adhesion between tube and/or ovary and the pelvic sidewall
Engage in minimal instrument handling of the tubes and ovaries to avoid traumatic exfoliation of cells
Both ovaries and tubes should be placed in an endobag for retrieval from the pelvis
Both ovaries and tubes should be processed by sectioning and extensively examining the fimbriated end (SEE-FIM) protocol
If occult malignancy or serous tubal intraepithelial carcinoma (STIC) is identified, provide referral to a gynecologic oncologist
The prevention benefits of salpingectomy alone are not yet proven. If considered, the fallopian tube from the fimbria to its insertion into the uterus should be removed. In addition, the fallopian tube should be processed and assessed as described above. The concern for risk-reducing salpingectomy alone is that patients are still at risk for developing ovarian cancer. In addition, in premenopausal patients, oophorectomy reduces the risk of developing breast cancer, but the magnitude is uncertain

NCCN Clinical Practice Guidelines in Oncology (Ovarian Cancer)

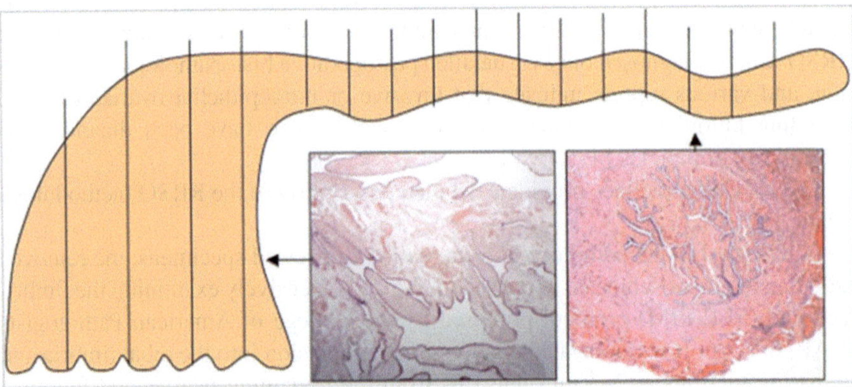

Fig. 1.1 Sectioning and extensively examining the fimbriated end (SEE-FIM) protocol. This protocol entails amputation and longitudinal sectioning of the infundibulum and fimbrial segment (distal 2 cm) to allow maximal exposure of the tubal plicae

81% of fallopian tube cancers that develop in patients with HBOC are HGSCs [18]. In the GOG0199 study, owing to the absence of an established protocol for the detailed histopathological examination of the fallopian tube removed during RRSO, the rate of discovery of abnormal findings, such as STIC, was low [14]. When RRSO is performed, the resected specimens were processed according to the SEE-FIM protocol proposed by CAP, and p53 and Ki-67 immunostaining was conducted thereafter. The purpose of these studies was to identify p53 signatures, such as p53

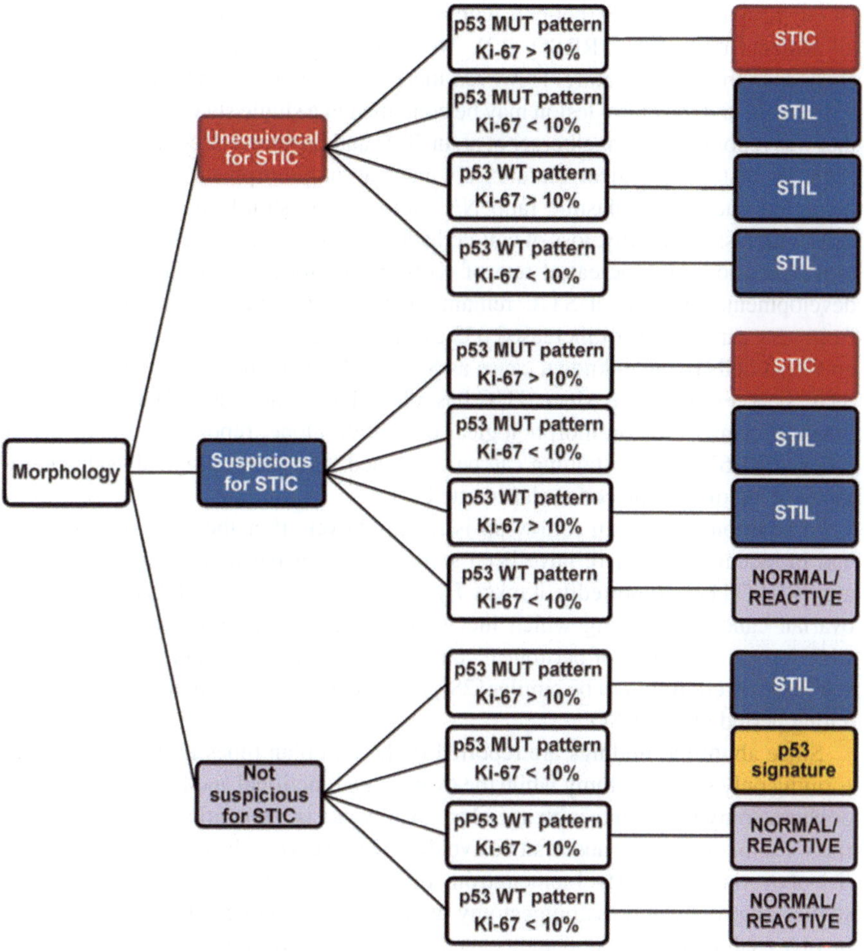

Fig. 1.2 Algorithm for the diagnosis of STIC. Foci showing a Ki-67 labeling index >10% are considered Ki-67 high, whereas a Ki-67 labeling index of <10% is considered low. Diffuse moderate-to-strong expression of p53 in >75% of at least 12 epithelial cells (with or without intervening ciliated cells) or complete absence of staining has been shown to be compatible with a *TP53* mutation either missense or nonsense (p53 MUT versus p53WT pattern in algorithm) [17]

overexpression and low Ki-67 positivity, albeit in morphologically benign nonciliary cells from the fallopian tubes of patients with HBOC, as proposed by Crum et al.; p53 signatures in tissues also suggest that it is a precursor lesion for STIC [19]. Although it is not considered necessary in routine medical practice, it is regarded as a diagnostic aid in HBOC diagnosis and treatment [20]. Furthermore, cells reportedly detach from the STIC formed in the tubal fimbria and engraft on the nearby ovarian surface, and STIC cells proliferate to form a mass, thereby leading to the development of HGSC [21–23]. Evolutionary analysis by laser capture microdissection also reported that the p53 signature and STIC of tubal lesions are precursors to

HGSC [24]. Furthermore, patients with p53 signature reportedly account for 25% of all patients undergoing RRSO [12]. We believe that it is necessary to monitor changes in the p53 signature. However, there are limitations in the SEE-FIM protocol as well, and the entire lesion may be contained in a single slice. STIC is a concept that was reported by Kingelberger et al. in 2007 and primarily occurs in tubal fimbria [25]. Its histopathological features are nuclear polymorphism, distinct nucleoli, increased nucleo-cytoplasmic ratio N/C ratio, pseudostratification of non-ciliated cells with loss of polarity, loss of cell-cell adhesion (detachment into the lumen), p53 overexpression, and increased rate of Ki-67 positivity (>15%) [26]. Although the developmental process of STIC remains unclear, Kurman et al. identified lesions from very early stages of increased p53 expression caused by DNA damage to tubal epithelial cells by an unknown cause as STIL and considered them as precursors to STIC [27]. Furthermore, since STIC has a low diagnostic concordance rate among diagnosticians based on morphological evaluation alone, reportedly, the results of p53 and Ki-67 immunostaining can be combined with morphological evaluation to increase the diagnostic concordance rate [17].

In addition, long-term follow-up is required even after the diagnosis of STIC, and in recent years, there have been some reports of peritoneal cancer diagnosis after RRSO [12]. Reportedly, it takes 7 years from the onset of STIC to the onset of ovarian cancer, following which metastasis progresses rapidly [24]. Since there were reports and cases of peritoneal cancer detection after 7 years or more, and tissue clones were found to be similar [28], it is necessary to continue surveillance for a long period after RRSO.

Since abnormal findings are reported in the fallopian tubes in many cases, performing only salpingectomy while the ovaries are functional and following this with oophorectomy in patients with age close to 50 years is a potential method to reduce risks. Premature menopause can be avoided by preserving the ovaries, although the risk of ovarian cancer development from the ovarian epithelium remains. Prospective studies on prophylactic salpingectomy with delayed oophorectomy (PSDO), which involves salpingectomy in patients aged 40 years and awaiting oophorectomy until the age of 50 years, have been initiated [29, 30]. However, some reports show that only 40%–60% of HGSCs develop from the fallopian tubes [25, 31], and NCCN guidelines [2, 9] have not yet confirmed the protective effect of salpingectomy alone; hence, it is not considered a standard treatment for risk reduction. As salpingectomy performed without other procedures cannot be expected to allay concerns of ovarian cancer development and reduce breast cancer risks, further discussions are needed. Currently, a multicenter, prospective, non-randomized study of PSDO in BRCA mutation carriers is underway [32].

After RRSO, 1%–4.3% residual risk for a primary peritoneal carcinoma has been reported in some studies. An analysis of 36 carriers of a BRCA1/2 variant who developed peritoneal carcinomatosis following RRSO showed that 86% were carriers of a *BRCA1* variant specifically [33]. When comparing to 113 carriers of a *BRCA1/2* variant who did not develop peritoneal carcinomatosis following RRSO, females who eventually developed peritoneal carcinomatosis were older at the time of RRSO ($P = 0.025$) and had a greater percentage of serous tubal intraepithelial carcinoma (STIC) in their RRSO specimen ($P < 0.001$), supporting the removal of the fallopian tubes as part of the risk-reducing procedure. A systematic review and individual patient data meta-analysis including 17 studies and 3121 patients showed that STIC at RRSO was strongly associated with increased risk of peritoneal carcinomatosis (HR, 33.9; 95% CI, 15.6–73.9; $P < 0.001$) [34].

On a different issue, there is no certain view on the treatment of a lesion found in the fallopian tubes after RRSO. While obvious fallopian tube cancer is treated according to the guidelines, there is no set view on STIC and other lesions. Although most patients are followed up for a long period of time [35], some of the cases collected by JOHBOC were treated with chemotherapy after STIC.

With the partial approval of diagnostic and therapeutic approaches for HBOC under insurance, the diagnosis rate for these conditions has improved owing to the increased use of genetic counseling and the expanded provision of information. In addition, the need for RRSO has permeated, and currently, several patients are undergoing RRSO. Moreover, it is necessary to educate patients regarding ovarian cancer at the time of breast cancer diagnosis. Laparoscopic RRSO is a procedure that can be conducted safely, but long-term follow-up is needed to monitor the postoperative development of peritoneal cancer and adverse events. Furthermore, a more detailed histopathological diagnosis will allow for the identification of small abnormalities in the fallopian tube. Considering the significance of such lesions, we believe that long-term treatment information and follow-up are of paramount importance.

References

1. Siegel RL, Miller KD, Jemal A. Cancer statistics, 2019. CA Cancer J Clin. 2019;69:7–34.
2. NCCN Guidelines insights: genetic/familial high-risk assessment: breast, ovarian, and pancreatic, Version 3.2024.
3. Kauff ND, Satagopan JM, Robson ME, et al. Risk-reducing salpingo-oophorectomy in women with a BRCA1 or BRCA2 mutation. N Engl J Med. 2002;346:1609–15.
4. Rebbeck TR, Lynch HT, Neuhausen SL, et al. Prophylactic oophorectomy in carriers of BRCA1 or BRCA2 mutations. N Engl J Med. 2002;346:1616–22.
5. Finch A, Beiner M, Lubinski J, et al. Salpingo-oophorectomy and the risk of ovarian, fallopian tube, and peritoneal cancers in women with a BRCA1 or BRCA2 Mutation. JAMA. 2006;296:185–92.
6. Domchek SM, Friebel TM, Neuhausen SL, et al. Mortality after bilateral salpingo-oophorectomy in BRCA1 and BRCA2 mutation carriers: a prospective cohort study. Lancet Oncol. 2006;7:223–9.
7. Rebbeck TR, Kauff ND, Domchek SM. Meta-analysis of risk reduction estimates associated with risk-reducing salpingo-oophorectomy in BRCA1 or BRCA2 mutation carriers. J Natl Cancer Inst. 2009;101:80–7.
8. Domchek SM, Friebel TM, Singer CF, et al. Association of risk-reducing surgery in BRCA1 or BRCA2 mutation carriers with cancer risk and mortality. JAMA. 2010;304:967–75.
9. Kauff ND, Domchek SM, Friebel TM, et al. Risk-reducing salpingo-oophorectomy for the prevention of BRCA1- and BRCA2-associated breast and gynecologic cancer: a multicenter, prospective study. J Clin Oncol. 2008;26:1331–7.

10. Nomura H, Sekine M, Yokoyama S, et al. Clinical background and outcomes of risk-reducing salpingo-oophorectomy for hereditary breast and ovarian cancers in Japan. Int J Clin Oncol. 2019;24:1105–10.
11. Marchetti C, De Felice F, Palaia I, et al. Risk-reducing salpingo-oophorectomy: a meta-analysis on impact on ovarian cancer risk and all cause mortality in BRCA 1 and BRCA 2 mutation carriers. BMC Womens Health. 2014;14:150.
12. Stanciu PI, Ind TEJ, Barton DPJ, et al. Development of peritoneal carcinoma in women diagnosed with serous tubal intraepithelial carcinoma (STIC) following risk-reducing salpingo-oophorectomy (RRSO). J Ovarian Res. 2019;12:50.
13. Nomura H, Ikki A, Fusegi A, et al. Clinical and pathological outcomes of risk-reducing salpingo-oophorectomy for Japanese women with hereditary breast and ovarian cancer. Int J Clin Oncol. 2021;26:2331–7.
14. Sherman ME, Piedmonte M, Mai PL, et al. Pathologic findings at risk-reducing salpingo-oophorectomy: primary results from Gynecologic Oncology Group Trial GOG-0199. J Clin Oncol. 2014;32:3275–83.
15. Crum CP, Drapkin R, Miron A, et al. The distal fallopian tube: a new model for pelvic serous carcinogenesis. Curr Opin Obstet Gynecol. 2007;19:3–9.
16. Medeiros F, Muto MG, Lee Y, et al. The tubal fimbria is a preferred site for early adenocarcinoma in women with familial ovarian cancer syndrome. Am J Surg Pathol. 2006;30:230–6.
17. Visvanathan K, Vang R, Shaw P, et al. Diagnosis of serous tubal intraepithelial carcinoma based on morphologic and immunohistochemical features: a reproducibility study. Am J Surg Pathol. 2011;35:1766–75.
18. Carlson JW, Miron A, Jarboe EA, et al. Serous tubal intraepithelial carcinoma: its potential role in primary peritoneal serous carcinoma and serous cancer prevention. J Clin Oncol. 2008;26:4160–5.
19. Lee Y, Miron A, Drapkin R, et al. A candidate precursor to serous carcinoma that originates in the distal fallopian tube. J Pathol. 2007;211:26–35.
20. Leonhardt K, Einenkel J, Sohr S, Engeland K, Horn LC. p53 signature and serous tubal in-situ carcinoma in cases of primary tubal and peritoneal carcinomas and serous borderline tumors of the ovary. Int J Gynecol Pathol. 2011;30:417–24.
21. Piek JM, van Diest PJ, Zweemer RP, et al. Dysplastic changes in prophylactically removed fallopian tubes of women predisposed to developing ovarian cancer. J Pathol. 2001;195:451–6.
22. Colgan TJ, Murphy J, Cole DE, Narod S, Rosen B. Occult carcinoma in prophylactic oophorectomy specimens: prevalence and association with BRCA germline mutation status. Am J Surg Pathol. 2001;25:1283–9.
23. Kurman RJ, Shih I. The origin and pathogenesis of epithelial ovarian cancer: a proposed unifying theory. Am J Surg Pathol. 2010;34:433–43.
24. Labidi-Galy SI, Papp E, Hallberg D, et al. High grade serous ovarian carcinomas originate in the fallopian tube. Nat Commun. 2017;8:1093.
25. Kindelberger DW, Lee Y, Miron A, et al. Intraepithelial carcinoma of the fimbria and pelvic serous carcinoma: evidence for a causal relationship. Am J Surg Pathol. 2007;31:161–9.
26. Kurman RJ, Carcangiu ML, Herrington CS, Young RH. WHO classification of tumor of female reproductive organs. ARC 2014.
27. Gross AL, Kurman RJ, Vang R, Shih I, Visvanathan K. Precursor lesions of high-grade serous ovarian carcinoma: morphological and molecular characteristics. J Oncol. 2010;2010:126295.
28. Blok F, Dasgupta S, Dinjens WNM, Roes EM, van Beekhuizen HJ, Ewing-Graham PC. Retrospective study of a 16 year cohort of BRCA1 and BRCA2 carriers presenting for RRSO: prevalence of invasive and in-situ carcinoma, with follow-up. Gynecol Oncol. 2019;153:326–34.
29. Holman LL, Friedman S, Daniels MS, Sun CC, Lu KH. Acceptability of prophylactic salpingectomy with delayed oophorectomy as risk-reducing surgery among BRCA mutation carriers. Gynecol Oncol. 2014;133:283–6.

30. Kwon JS, Tinker A, Pansegrau G, et al. Prophylactic salpingectomy and delayed oophorectomy as an alternative for BRCA mutation carriers. Obstet Gynecol. 2013;121:14–24.
31. Przybycin CG, Kurman RJ, Ronnett BM, Shih I, Vang R. Are all pelvic (nonuterine) serous carcinomas of tubal origin? Am J Surg Pathol. 2010;34:1407–16.
32. Harmsen MG, Arts-de Jong M, Hoogerbrugge N, et al. Early salpingectomy (TUbectomy) with delayed oophorectomy to improve quality of life as alternative for risk-reducing salpingo-oophorectomy in BRCA1/2 mutation carriers (TUBA study): a prospective non-randomised multicentre study. BMC Cancer. 2015;15:593.
33. Harmsen MG, Piek JMJ, Bulten J, et al. Peritoneal carcinomatosis after risk-reducing surgery in BRCA1/2 mutation carriers. Cancer. 2018;124:952–9.
34. Steenbeek MP, van Bommel MHD, Bulten J, et al. Risk of peritoneal carcinomatosis after risk-reducing salpingo-oophorectomy: a systematic review and individual patient data meta-analysis. J Clin Oncol. 2022;40:1879–91.
35. Saccardi C, Zovato S, Spagnol G, et al. Efficacy of risk-reducing salpingo-oophorectomy in BRCA1-2 variants and clinical outcomes of follow-up in patients with isolated serous tubal intraepithelial carcinoma (STIC). Obstet Gynecol. 2021;163:364–70.

Chapter 2
Prostate/Pancreatic Cancer in HBOC

Koji Nishino

Abstract Individuals with *BRCA1/2* pathogenic germline variants are at increased risk of developing prostate and pancreatic cancer as well as breast and ovarian cancer, although the names of disease "hereditary breast and ovarian cancer (HBOC)" might not suggest. Diagnosis of pancreatic cancer at early stage is extremely difficult, but recommended surveillance for those with *BRCA1/2* variants has been suggested for both prostate and pancreatic cancer. Overwhelmingly, HBOC is found to be first diagnosed in patients with breast or ovarian cancer within their families. When we find a HBOC patient, we must remember that prostate and pancreatic cancer are also HBOC-related cancers, and it is necessary to help share this information among their family members, including "men."

Keywords Prostate cancer · PSA surveillance · Pancreatic cancer · MRCP/EUS surveillance

2.1 Introduction

The name "hereditary breast and ovarian cancer (HBOC)" may not be an appropriate description of the disease. *BRCA1/2* pathogenic germline variants(PGV)are present regardless of gender, and they also increase the risk of developing pancreatic and prostate cancer. In Japan, this awareness is not widespread enough, which is why *BRCA1/2* germline testing tends not to be done for appropriate subjects, especially in male. In this chapter, the basic information on pancreatic and prostate cancer are described that may not be fully understood from the disease name "HBOC," but for which the risk of morbidity is definitely increased in the presence of *BRCA1/2* PGV.

K. Nishino (✉)
Department of Familial and Hereditary Oncology (Obstetrics and Gynecology), Niigata University Graduate School of Medical and Dental Sciences, Niigata City, Japan
e-mail: knishino@med.niigata-u.ac.jp

A. Sakurai et al. (eds.), *Practical Guide to Hereditary Breast and Ovarian Cancer II*, https://doi.org/10.1007/978-981-96-4329-5_2

2.2 Prostate Cancer

2.2.1 *Epidemiology; Morbidity, Mortality, and Survival*

In Japan, 92,021 males were diagnosed with prostate cancer (PC) in 2018 [1]; this is the first highest number of cancer cases among men. On the other hand, the number of deaths is low at 12544 [1], and the disease is considered to have a low mortality rate. PC is also common in the elderly male and with a favorable prognosis, with 5-year survival rate of 100% for early disease, 99.2% for locally advanced, and 53.4% for disease with distant metastases. One of the characteristics of PC is the option of "active surveillance" without any invasive treatment, depending on age or stage, especially when expected life expectancy is short, less than 10 years [2].

2.2.2 *Screening and Diagnosis*

There is an effective screening method for PC, whether it is hereditary or not. Prostate-specific antigen (PSA) is a specific tumor marker that is elevated in PC, with a reference value of 0–4 ng/ml. In cases of abnormally high levels of PSA, a definitive diagnosis by transrectal prostate biopsy may be considered. PSA screening for PC is currently recommended in Japan from the age of 50 years, with a cut-off value of 4 ng/ml [3]. On the other hand, PSA can also be elevated in benign prostatic hyperplasia and inflammation of the prostate and can also lead to overdiagnosis, but it is an accessible testing method with relatively low cost and is easy to access [4].

2.2.3 BRCA-*Positive Prostate Cancer*

Males with *BRCA1/2* PGV are more susceptible to PC. Of all, 1–2% are considered *BRCA*-positive PC. The risk is higher for those with *BRCA2* PGV, with 27% developing PC by age 75 and 60% by age 85(OR; 4.45, 95%CI; 2.99–6.61). On the other hand, males with *BRCA1* PGV are 21% more likely to develop PC by age 75 and 29% by age 85(OR; 2.35, 95%CI; 1.43–3.38) [5] (Fig. 2.1).

In addition, *BRCA*-positive PC has a poorer prognosis than sporadic cancers [6], both in local and in advanced cases with distant metastases. This is due to carrying many poor prognostic factors such as Gleason score > 8, T3/4, lymph node, and distant metastases, which is why *BRCA*-positive PC is not indicated for active surveillance, and proactive therapeutic intervention is recommended [7] (Fig. 2.2).

PSA surveillance is also effective for *BRCA*-positive PC. The IMPACT study [8] of 3027 males aged 40–69 (including 919 with *BRCA1* PGV, 909 with *BRCA2*) followed by annual PSA surveillance for 3 years, with prostate biopsy when the PSA

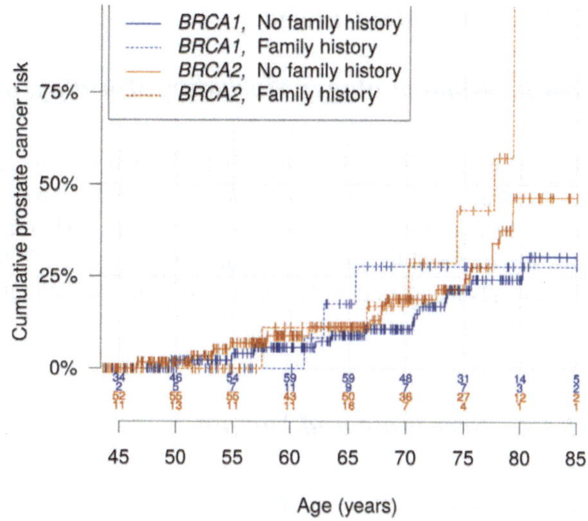

Fig. 2.1 Risk of developing prostate cancer according to age and *BRCA* status. (Nyberg et al. [5])
The risk is higher for those with *BRCA2* PGV, with 27% developing prostate cancer by age 75 and 60% by age 85(OR; 4.45, 95%CI; 2.99–6.61). Males with *BRCA1* PGV are 21% more likely to develop prostate cancer by age 75 and 29% by age 85 (OR; 2.35, 95%CI; 1.43–3.38)

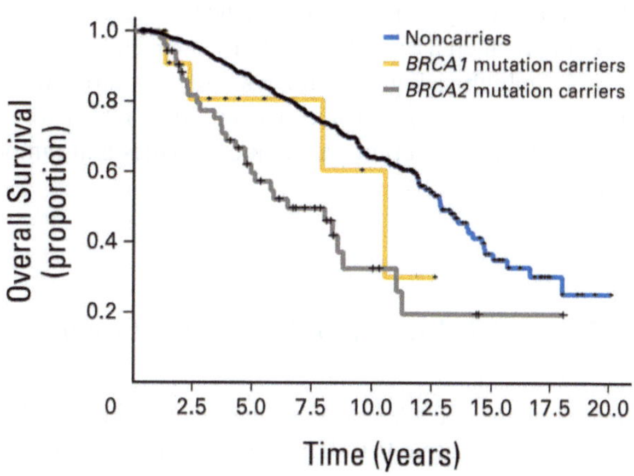

Fig. 2.2 Survival curves of Prostate cancer according to BRCA status. (Castro et al. [7])
Overall survival outcome of prostate cancer with BRCA1/2 PGV is worse than sporadic cancers because they have many poor prognostic factors

levels exceed 3 ng/ml. As a result, 527 males had PSA levels above 3, and 357 biopsies were performed, of which 112 were diagnosed with prostate cancer (including 31 with *BRCA1* PGV, 47 with *BRCA2*). Males with *BRCA2* PGV were associated with a significantly higher incidence of PC, lower age of onset, and more highly malignant tumor with poorer pathological risk factors. On the other hand, male with *BRCA1* PGV only had these trends and no statistically significant differences. Based on these findings, PSA surveillance for *BRCA*-positive PC is currently recommended in Japan from the age of 40 years, with a cut-off value of 3 ng/ml; both are more young or strict than for sporadic cases [9].

2.3 Pancreatic Cancer

2.3.1 *Epidemiology; Morbidity, Mortality, and Survival*

In Japan, 21,559 males and 20,880 females were diagnosed with pancreatic cancer(PaC)in 2018 [1]. In contrast to PC, PaC's prognosis is extremely poor, and many cases are diagnosed at an advanced stage when curative surgical resection is already impossible, and 5-year survival rate is 42.1% for early disease, 12.4% for locally advanced, and 1.8% for disease with distant metastases.

2.3.2 *Screening and Diagnosis*

In contrast to PC, there is unfortunately no effective screening algorithm for early detection of PaC. On the other hand, it is also thought that early detection rates may be increased by performing enhanced CT, enhanced MRI (magnetic resonance cholangiopancreatography (MRCP), and endoscopic ultrasonography (EUS) for people in high-risk groups for PaC, such as those with a family history, complications of diabetes or chronic pancreatitis, or a history of smoking, as well as for people with high serum pancreatic enzymes and tumor markers(CA19–9, Span-1, and DUPAN-2) [10].

2.3.3 BRCA-*Positive Pancreatic Cancer*

People with *BRCA1/2* PGV are more susceptible to PaC. Of all, 3–4% are considered *BRCA*-positive PaC. The risk is higher for those with *BRCA2* PGV, with 2–7% developing PaC in lifetime, and 1–3% with *BRCA1* PGV [11].

The International Cancer of the Pancreas Screening (CAPS) Consortium presents a program of 55 recommendations on management guidelines for people at high risk of PaC (with certain genetic variants or family history). Among them are (1) individuals with *BRCA1/2* PGV with at least one first-degree relative with PaC, (2) individuals with *BRCA2* PGV with at least two PaC patients in their family tree, should be subjects to have some surveillance [12]. Although MRCP and EUS are highly recommended as the actual surveillance methods in this recommendation, no details are given on the age at which the tests should be started or how the two methods should be combined. Canto et al. [13] reported that nine of ten PaC detected by EUS/MRI/CT surveillance were curatively resectable and 85% survived 3 years, suggesting that these PaC surveillance may have a certain prognostic value (Fig. 2.3).

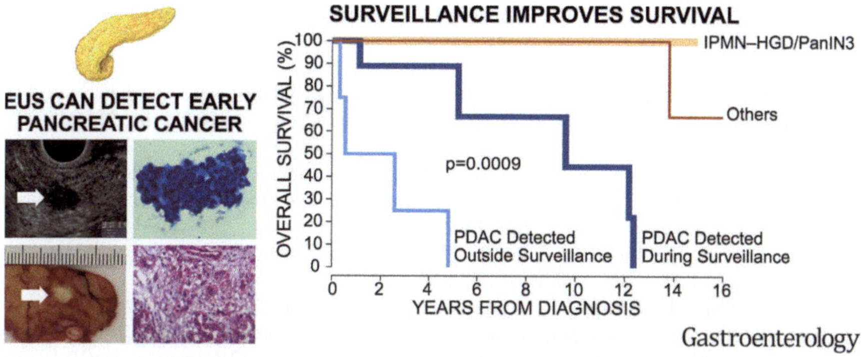

Fig. 2.3 Potential for improving survival of pancreatic cancer by surveillance. (Canto et al. [13]) Nine of 10 pancreatic cancer patients detected by EUS/MRI/CT surveillance were curatively resectable and 85% survived 3 years

Based on these findings, PaC surveillance by MRI or EUS is recommended for individuals with *BRCA1/2* PGV with a family history of PaC in at least one first-degree relative [9]. Although these surveillances could detect PaC at an early stage when curative resection is possible, they are expensive and complicated methods and cannot be performed as easily as PSA surveillance. Actually, there are very few facilities in Japan that can perform these examinations, and it is difficult to perform under Japanese insurance system.

2.4 Conclusion

Individuals with *BRCA1/2* pathogenic germline variants are at increased risk of developing prostate cancer (male) and pancreatic cancer (both sexes), and the risk of morbidity is higher in case with *BRCA2* PGV than with *BRCA1* in both malignancies.

Surveillance by serum PSA testing for prostate cancer is recommended, and EUS/MRI for pancreatic cancer is considered for individuals with *BRCA1/2* PGV.

Above all, the awareness that "prostate and pancreatic cancer are HBOC-associated cancers" needs to be widely shared among all medical doctors and patients, regardless of gender.

References

1. Cancer Statistics. Cancer Information Service, National Cancer Center, Japan (National Cancer Registry, Ministry of Health, Labour and Welfare).
2. Clinical Practice Guideline for Prostate Cancer 2016, The Japanese Urological Association, Medical Review Co.

3. Screening Guideline for Prostate Cancer 2018, The Japanese Urological Association, Medical Review Co.
4. https://www.urol.or.jp/
5. Nyberg T, et al. Prostate cancer risks for male BRCA1 and BRCA2 mutation carriers: a prospective cohort study. Eur Urol. 2020;77(1):24–35. https://doi.org/10.1016/j.eururo.2019.08.025. Epub 2019 Sept 6
6. Na R, et al. Germline mutations in ATM and BRCA1/2 distinguish risk for lethal and indolent prostate cancer and are associated with early age at death. Eur Urol. 2017;71(5):740–7. https://doi.org/10.1016/j.eururo.2016.11.033. Epub 2016 Dec 15
7. Castro E, et al. Germline BRCA mutations are associated with higher risk of nodal involvement, distant metastasis, and poor survival outcomes in prostate cancer. J Clin Oncol. 2013;31(14):1748–57. https://doi.org/10.1200/JCO.2012.43.1882. Epub 2013 Apr 8
8. Page EC, et al. Interim results from the IMPACT study: evidence for prostate-specific antigen screening in BRCA2 mutation carriers. Eur Urol. 2019;76(6):831–42. https://doi.org/10.1016/j.eururo.2019.08.019. Epub 2019 Sep 16
9. Guidelines for Diagnosis and Treatment of Hereditary Breast and Ovarian Cancer 2021, Japanese Organization of Hereditary Breast and Ovarian Cancer(JOHOBC), Kanehara-shuppan Co.
10. Clinical Practice Guideline for Pancreatic Cancer 2019, Japan pancreas society, Kanehara-shuppan Co.
11. Mizukami K, et al. Genetic characterization of pancreatic cancer patients and prediction of carrier status of germline pathogenic variants in cancer-predisposing genes. EBioMedicine. 2020;60:103033. https://doi.org/10.1016/j.ebiom.2020.103033. Epub 2020 Sep 24
12. Goggins M, et al. Management of patients with increased risk for familial pancreatic cancer: updated recommendations from the international cancer of the pancreas screening (CAPS) consortium. Gut. 2020;69(1):7–17. https://doi.org/10.1136/gutjnl-2019-319352. Epub 2019 Oct 31
13. Canto MI, et al. Risk of neoplastic progression in individuals at high risk for pancreatic cancer undergoing long-term surveillance. Gastroenterology. 2018;155(3):740–751.e2. https://doi.org/10.1053/j.gastro.2018.05.035.

Chapter 3
Regional Collaboration for Comprehensive HBOC Care

Narumi Harada-Shoji

Abstract The number of *BRCA1/2* carriers in Japan is expected to increase, and there is an urgent need to respond to the rapid advances in genetic medicine. However, there is a shortage of Japanese Organization of Hereditary Breast and Ovarian Cancer (JOHBOC)-certified facilities and limited availability of physicians, nurses, and certified genetic counselors offering genetic medicine. It is, therefore, essential to optimize the use of current resources and to train the personnel who will provide genetic medicine in the future. JOHBOC-certified facilities are located in urban areas in the Tohoku region, while some areas lack such certified facilities. The Tohoku region is strengthening cooperation between prefectures and utilizing existing resources in genetic medicine, taking into account factors such as long distances between cities and inadequate public transport. In addition, some facilities in various areas offer telemedicine services that eliminate the need for patients to physically visit a hospital. However, some medical professionals perceive genetic medicine as a psychological and physical burden, which requires the implementation of a comprehensive education system and the expansion of genetic medicine to ensure universal participation. Efforts should be made to achieve parity in the provision of appropriate healthcare systems for *BRCA1/2* carriers, to ensure that they can live in a society where they have equal peace of mind.

Keywords HBOC care · HBOC practice · Regional collaboration · Human resources and shared decision making (SDM)

N. Harada-Shoji (✉)
Department of Breast and Endocrine Surgical Oncology, Tohoku University Graduate School of Medicine, Sendai, Japan
e-mail: narumi.harada.a3@tohoku.ac.jp

A. Sakurai et al. (eds.), *Practical Guide to Hereditary Breast and Ovarian Cancer II*, https://doi.org/10.1007/978-981-96-4329-5_3

Abbreviations

HBOC	Hereditary breast and ovarian cancer
CGC	Certified genetic counselor
JOHBOC	Japanese Organization of Hereditary Breast and Ovarian Cancer
BRCA1/2 carriers	*BRCA1/2* pathogenic variant carriers
ABGC	American Board of Genetic Counselling
JSGO	Japan Society of Gynecologic Oncology
CNS-GN	Clinical Nurse Specialist in Genetic Nursing
MRI	Magnetic resonance imaging
DKG	German Cancer Society
GC-HBOC	German Consortium for Hereditary Breast and Ovarian Cancer
C-MOnGene	Collaborative Model in OncoGenetics

3.1 Introduction

Approximately 250,000 to 620,000 people in Japan have pathological mutations in *BRCA1* or *BRCA2*, which means that the number of people with hereditary breast and ovarian cancer (HBOC), including those who have not yet been diagnosed, is likely to increase. When a genetic test result indicates a pathological variant, it is essential to provide appropriate medical intervention. In the field of HBOC diagnosis, the main objective is not only to perform a genetic test but also to establish an effective follow-up system to contribute to the secondary prevention of cancer. For breast and ovarian cancer patients diagnosed with HBOC, surveillance and risk-reducing surgery are already available through the insurance system. As the diagnosis of HBOC involves genetic testing, professional genetic counseling by a clinical geneticist and a certified genetic counselor (CGC) is essential from before the test to understanding the results. Once diagnosed, HBOC services need to provide not only treatment for each type of cancer but also monitoring when the disease has not yet developed and support for family members who carry pathological variants, in a comprehensive manner, while sharing details of medical treatment through ongoing conferences. Organized care for HBOC requires input from a variety of disciplines and requires local collaboration to ensure that patients receive optimal HBOC care regardless of the area. By focusing on the involvement of multiple experts and organizations within an area, collaborative models can provide higher quality, more specialized care. These collaborations include aspects such as databases, telemedicine systems, and guidelines used by health care facilities.

This chapter describes the current status and challenges of HBOC medical collaborations in the context of Japanese society, with a focus on the Tohoku region. It then analyses partnership approaches in other countries and identifies directions for improving HBOC care in partnership with regions.

3.2 Current Status and Problems in Japan Regarding HBOC Care Coordination

As shown in Table 3.1, the Japanese Organization of Hereditary Breast and Ovarian Cancer (JOHBOC) has a core facility, affiliated facilities, and cooperating facilities for HBOC care in each district (a list of requirements for accreditation of each facility is available on the JOHBOC's website: https: //johboc.jp/gaiyou/regulations/shisetsu_ks/). The management system has been established to ensure that *BRCA1/2* pathogenic variant carriers (*BRCA1/2* carriers) receive appropriate medical care, taking account into consideration their place of residence and other factors. On the other

Table 3.1 Certified facility requirements and numbers of facilities in the region

Facility certification requirements *1	**Core facility**	**Collaborating facility**	**Supporting facility**		
Clinical Genetic Specialist	◎	○			
Certified Genetic Counselor	△				
Breast Specialist	◎	○	○		
Gynecologic Oncology Specialist	◎				
HBOC Genetic Testing Implementation	◎	◎			
Breast Cancer Surveillance	◎	○	○		
Gynecologic Surveillance	◎				
RRM	◎	○			
RRSO	◎				
HBOC Seminar	◎	◎	◎		
HBOC Conference	◎	◎			
Patient Registry	◎	◎			
Cooperation with Core Facilities for Comprehensive Medical Care		◎	◎		
◎: Required, △: Preferred ○: Either required					
Region	**Core facility**	**Collaborating facility**	**Supporting facility**	**Total**	**Population *2**
Hokkaido	3	1	2	6	53M
Tohoku	4	3	2	9	87M
Kantou	20	6	26	52	433M
Chubu	19	5	28	52	230M
Kinki	13	7	14	34	205M
Chugoku	7	6	19	32	73M
Shikoku	2	4	4	10	37M
Kyushu and Okinawa	3	1	2	6	140M

*1: https://johboc.jp/
*2: https://www.stat.go.jp/data/jinsui/index.html

hand, in a national survey on the coordination of HBOC care [1], it was clear that both medical care providers and *BRCA1/2* carriers face many problems, such as the following: First, the issue of inadequate pre-referral education was recognized as a problem. There are significant differences in the functions and roles of medical facilities, with some facilities lacking the capacity to offer advanced genetic testing and genetic counseling. In addition, each facility requires an individual coordination system, which poses a challenge in establishing standardized regulations. In addition, the genetic counseling system is complex, making regional cooperation difficult. There are also concerns about human resource constraints as the number of referrals from collaborating centers increases. Identifying the appropriate time to refer patients to core facilities is a challenge, and there is a lack of opportunities to engage with collaborating facilities. *BRCA1/2* carriers may not be able to undergo genetic testing if the distance to the core facility exceeds a certain threshold. Therefore, although genetic medicine is advancing rapidly following the introduction of insurance coverage for HBOC care, the existing system of medical care is still inadequate.

3.3 Personnel Resources and Burden Related to Medical Treatment

Human resources such as genetic counselors involved in genetic counseling, physicians in units providing surveillance and risk-reducing surgery, and nurses and psychologists involved in shared decision making (SDM) are also essential for the coordination of HBOC care. Genetic counseling generally refers to the provision of information and psychosocial support for genetic disorders. In the USA, training for "genetic counselors" has been offered since 1970 in master's programs at graduate schools of public health and is accredited by the American Board of Genetic Counselling (ABGC). Upon completion of the training program and passing the certification examination, students are awarded CGC status. Data from 2018 shows that there are more than 4000 certified CGCs. Looking at other countries, there are approximately 900 genetic counselors in Cuba, 350 in Canada, 310 in the United Kingdom, and 220 in Australia/New Zealand, illustrating the different development of the genetic medicine profession in each country [2]. In Japan, genetic counseling in genetic medicine is considered a medical practice, and many institutions provide genetic counseling mainly through CGCs, clinical genetic specialists, and physicians in charge of medical departments or genetic counseling. In recent years, a system of CGCs has been established in Japan through joint accreditation by the Japanese Society of Genetic Counselling and the Japan Society of Human Genetics, and currently (April 2023) 356 people are certified as CGCs. However, the history of genetic counseling for cancer in Japan is still young, and it was only in the second half of the 1990s that it became a serious endeavor [3].

A survey conducted by the Japan Society of Gynecologic Oncology (JSGO) revealed the following psychological burdens for obstetricians and gynecologists in the management of HBOC [4]. While the use of poly (ADP-ribose) polymerase

(PARP) inhibitors and the use of *BRCA* gene testing as an adjunctive diagnosis were perceived as having a low psychological burden, the uninsured use of *BRCA* gene testing and the explanation and counseling of patients who have not yet developed the disease were perceived by many physicians as having a high psychological burden.

The uninsured provision of RRSO was also perceived as a significant psychological burden. These findings suggest that obstetricians and gynecologists face a great psychological burden in dealing with uninsured patients and providing treatment that is not covered by insurance, and that there is a need to strengthen the support system for medical personnel and to provide easy-to-understand explanatory materials for patients. In addition, a study by a group from the Japanese Breast Cancer Association is investigating the level of understanding of HBOC care among physicians and nurses involved in breast care, as well as the time and psychological burden associated with genetic medicine, and the results are awaited.

3.4 Problems in HBOC Care in the Tohoku Region

A survey conducted in April 2022 revealed that the Tohoku region has 11 CGCs and one Clinical Nurse Specialist in Genetic Nursing (CNS-GN) at 68 facilities accredited and affiliated with the Breast Cancer Society. However, despite this considerable presence, there is an undeniable shortage of personnel involved in HBOC care. As illustrated in Fig. 3.1, JOHBOC-accredited facilities are situated in urban areas within the Tohoku region, with no such facilities present in Akita Prefecture. In comparison to other regions, the distances between cities are greater, and the topography of the area necessitates that patients visit remote hospitals, which presents a physical disadvantage. A survey was conducted of CGCs, CNS-GNs, and certified breast cancer nurses in order to ascertain the current status of and problems with the HBOC care system in the Tohoku region. A total of 19 facilities were able to ascertain the current status of HBOC care. Of the 19 facilities surveyed, 11 (58%) were able to perform risk-reducing surgery under insurance coverage. The remaining facilities were unable to do so due to a lack of additional magnetic resonance imaging (MRI) scans or the absence of specialist physicians. Eight facilities (8/19, 42%) were able to perform risk-reducing surgery on patients who had not yet developed the disease. In the event that risk-reducing surgery could not be performed at their own institution, patients were referred to facilities that could perform the procedure through the Regional Coordination Office. In some cases, patients were referred to other prefectures. In Tohoku University Hospital, both the Department of Breast Surgery and the Department of Gynecology have established a system of regional cooperation specializing in HBOC. However, many respondents in other regions highlighted the lack of a substantial network as a significant challenge. In the Tohoku region, it is imperative to enhance interregional collaboration, taking into account the geographical constraints.

Tohoku University Hospital, a JOHBOC-certified core facility, has established an internal and external collaboration system with the objective of facilitating the

Fig. 3.1 The number of certified facilities in Tohoku (prefecture and population)

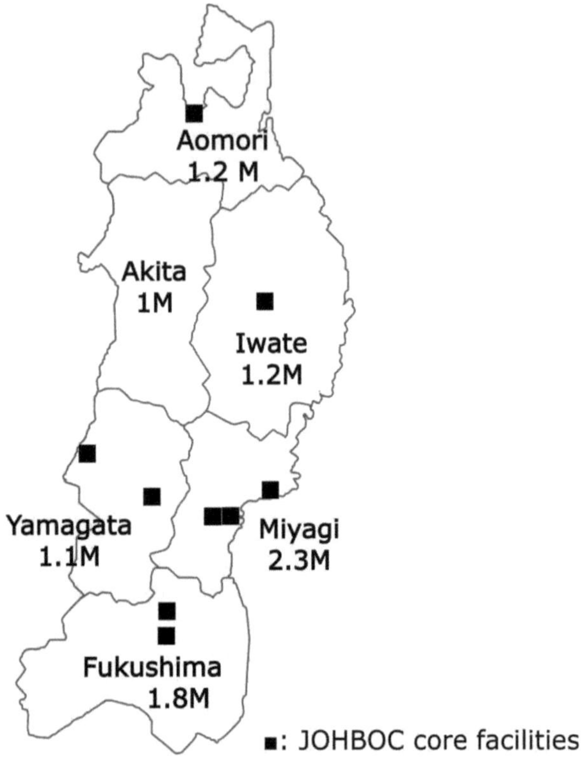

provision of optimal HBOC care. In addition, the three departments of Breast and Endocrine Surgery, Gynecology, and Genetics have established HBOC outpatient slots in each department to provide seamless in-hospital referrals for breast cancer/ovarian cancer surveillance, risk-reducing surgery, and genetic counseling. Furthermore, the Department of Plastic and Reconstructive Surgery and the Department of Diagnostic Radiology collaborate closely with regard to risk-reducing surgery and diagnostic imaging, respectively, and convene regular conferences. Individuals carrying the *BRCA1/2* carriers who request surveillance for pancreatic cancer are referred to the Department of Gastroenterology. For male *BRCA1/2* carriers who have not yet developed prostate cancer, the initial diagnosis involves monitoring prostate-specific antigen (PSA) levels, which is carried out by the Department of Breast and Endocrine Surgery. If the PSA level exceeds 3.0 ng/mL, the patient is then referred to the Department of Urology for further investigation. Furthermore, referrals from other medical institutions that are not suitable for risk-reducing surgery or genetic counseling are also managed through a regional cooperative framework for HBOC outpatients (Fig. 3.2).

In the challenging geographical conditions of the Tohoku region, where it is complicated to reach a JOHBOC-accredited institution, the CGC conducts visits to each hospital. The objective of these services is to provide genetic counseling and to create an accessible environment for *BRCA1/2* carriers who require genetic

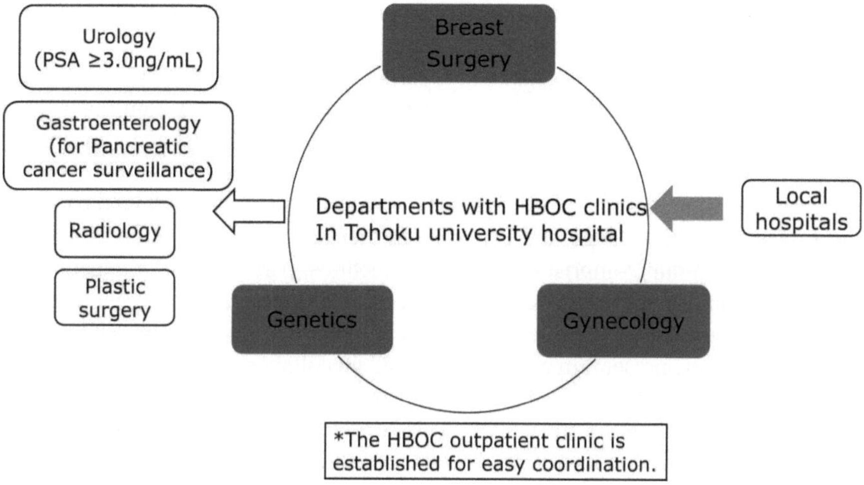

Fig. 3.2 HBOC care at Tohoku University

medical care. Furthermore, due to the limited availability of facilities for risk-reducing surgery, a collaborative approach has been adopted among hospitals to ensure the efficient delivery of the treatment and optimize the utilization of scarce human resources.

3.5 HBOC Care Collaboration Efforts in Other Countries

It is crucial to maintain a balance between the demand for quality medical care and the needs of patients in the supply of HBOC care. As previously stated, the demand for HBOC has increased rapidly in Japan since insurance coverage was implemented. It is therefore anticipated that the number of blood relatives tested will continue to rise in the future. In the USA, HBOC is estimated to affect more than one million individuals, necessitating the implementation of an appropriate system for the provision of genetic medicine [5]. The identification of HBOC requires not only the genetic testing of family members, a process known as ふ ま n testing or screening, but also companion diagnostic purpose for the use of PARP inhibitors. Additionally, factors such as recommendations for risk-reducing surgery and surveillance must be considered. The progression of technology and the reduction in costs have led to a shift in genetic testing practices. What was previously conducted as single-gene genetic testing has now evolved into multigene panel genomic testing [6, 7]. The accessibility of HBOC testing has increased, yet this has the potential to exacerbate existing health disparities. Patients, at-risk family members, and healthcare providers are confronted with numerous challenges, including the necessity for psychological support in the event of positive, negative, or indeterminate test results [8].

The German Cancer Society (DKG) has published a position paper addressing the challenges of cancer patient care in the era of genomic medicine. The German Consortium for Hereditary Breast and Ovarian Cancer (GC-HBOC) has incorporated these recommendations into its concept of care for at-risk families [9]. In 2015, a cross-disciplinary network of accredited centers for breast and gynecological cancer was established with the objective of developing an educational program for professional nurses and physicians. The objective of this network is to facilitate the exchange of knowledge and expertise in the field of genetic counseling. The educational program comprises face-to-face lectures, participation in genetic case conferences, and actual genetic counseling sessions. This ensured that genetic counseling and testing were provided in accordance with the most recent advances in knowledge. At the present time, the GC-HBOC, in collaboration with the DKG and with financial support from the Federal Ministry of Health, is engaged in the development of a unified online curriculum. This curriculum draws upon existing online lectures from the United Kingdom, the Netherlands, and Australia [10].

The C-MOnGene (Collaborative Model in OncoGenetics) study, conducted in Canada, resulted in the development of a "collaborative oncogenetic model." This model included the incorporation of genetic testing by nongenetic physicians and genetic specialists, group counseling, and coordination of medical institutions [11]. Over the course of the three-year implementation period, the number of patients receiving genetic counseling increased at a rate of 100% annually, demonstrating a significant and sustained growth in this area of patient care. Moreover, the mean interval between genetic counseling and the disclosure of test results was significantly reduced. Group counseling was demonstrated to be an efficacious method of improving participants' understanding of breast cancer risk and increasing their knowledge of breast cancer and genetics. It is proposed that this model will facilitate the delivery of efficient genetic counseling and *BRCA1/2* testing while also accelerating the practice of HBOC.

3.6 Current Practices and Challenges

Table 3.2 provides a summary of the challenges and proposed solutions for HBOC practice in Japan. The severe shortage of human resources in the field of genetic medicine represents a significant challenge to the provision of HBOC care in Japan. Genetic medicine, including genetic counseling, will need to be continuous, as risk reducing surgery and surveillance options are likely to change with life stage and changing circumstances. There will also be a need for genetic counseling even when genetic tests are negative, which will contribute to the shortage of human resources [12]. However, there is a paucity of precise data concerning the precise number of individuals required to achieve equilibrium between supply and demand. Prior to training medical personnel in genetic medicine, it is of utmost importance to initially enhance awareness of HBOC. It is anticipated that the significance of genetic medicine will increase in line with the acquisition of greater knowledge about it. It

Table 3.2 Problems and solutions in HBOC practice

	Problems	Solutions
1. Human resource shortage	Japan has a severe lack of resources for genetic medicine	Incorporate core genetic medicine knowledge into medical education and enhance awareness of HBOC
2. Leadership gap	Insufficient leaders to advocate for the advancement of genetic medicine	Provide leadership programs that educate and support leaders in genetic medicine
3. Education in program deficiency	Contemporary training programs for HBOC practitioners are insufficient	Implement continuous professional development through e-learning and regular seminars provided by JOHBOC, ensuring practitioners stay informed with the latest advancements
4, Geographical access limitations	Geographical limitations make genetic treatment difficult to obtain in places like Okinawa and Tohoku	Utilize telemedicine to boost accessibility in underserved areas and offer genetic counseling remotely
5. Psychosocial and economic burdens	The financial, social, and psychological costs associated with an HBOC diagnosis are rarely well addressed	Initiate comprehensive research to identify these burdens and develop tailored support systems
6. Physicians' lack of understanding of HBOC	Patients and physicians addressing breast and ovarian cancer may not have a good knowledge of HBOC, risk-reducing surgery, and surveillance	Conduct targeted surveys to identify knowledge gaps and deliver education tailored to the needs of healthcare providers and patients

is therefore vital that fundamental knowledge required is integrated into the medical curriculum during the study process [13].

Moreover, there is an evident dearth of leaders capable of disseminating genetic medicine. It is anticipated that CGC and CNS-GN will engage not only in clinical practice but also in research and education [14, 15]. Moreover, the shortage of genetic counselors in Japan is partly due to a lack of sufficient employment opportunities, while there is a shortage of human resources, and it is also important to raise the status of the profession [16]. However, a system that relies solely on genetic medicine specialists such as clinical geneticists and genetic counselors could 1 day collapse. In the future, it is imperative that all physicians, including those engaged in the provision of breast and gynecological care, assume a position at the threshold of genetic medicine and extend the scope of genetic medicine.

JOHBOC provides e-learning seminars for medical practitioners who are either in the initial stages of their careers or planning to become involved in HBOC practice (https://johboc.jp/kyoiku/e-learningseminar/). The seminars are designed to be highly convenient, with each session able to be taken in installments or repeated within the viewing institution. Furthermore, an update seminar for HBOC practitioners is provided to ensure practitioners remain up to date with the latest developments in HBOC practice. As previously indicated, online curricula have been conducted in Germany, the United Kingdom, the Netherlands, and Australia. The results of these studies have demonstrated high levels of satisfaction [17]. The satisfaction levels reported for online lectures are significantly higher than those reported for face-to-face lectures. This increased satisfaction can be attributed to the educators' routine guidance and the enhanced competence of the participants. Moreover, a distinct curriculum for nurses has been established in Germany to facilitate a multidisciplinary team approach [18, 19]. It is anticipated that a genetic medicine program for nurses will serve to disseminate genetic medicine throughout Japan.

While the enhancement of educational program will contribute to the securing of human resources, the creation of an environment in which *BRCA1/2* carriers can access genetic medicine is an equally important issue that requires resolution. As previously stated, the Tohoku region lacks the requisite infrastructure for genetic medicine, due to the limited number of genetic medicine facilities and the region's geographical conditions. According to data from the Ministry of Land, Infrastructure, Transport and Tourism, the average length of city pairs in the Tohoku region is approximately 28 km. The transportation system is also not fully advance as of Tokyo metropolitan area, and this hampers the clients to get access to the hospital that is offering genetic treatment. The situation is similar in Okinawa Prefecture, which has many remote islands, and this is an issue that needs to be addressed not only in the Tohoku region but also in Japan as a whole. As a solution to this problem, remote genetic counseling has been initiated at a limited number of medical institutions, taking advantage of the rapidly advancing online medical technology that has emerged since the COVID-19 pandemic, making genetic counseling available to people regardless of where they live, and playing a role in the spread of genetic medicine. This has made genetic counseling available to people regardless of their geographical location, thereby facilitating the dissemination of genetic medicine. Similar initiatives are being implemented in other countries. A multicenter study conducted at seven US hospitals evaluated the feasibility and impact of reporting genetic test results and providing genetic counseling to patients with Parkinson's disease. The findings indicated that both hospitals near the patient's place of residence and remote groups demonstrated higher levels of knowledge and satisfaction with genetic testing [20]. For genetic care to be effectively delivered, a well-developed genetic counseling system is required, and this is expected to increase in the future in Japan.

HBOC care is evolving toward a new phase; however, the psychosocial and economic implications of a diagnosis have yet to be fully elucidated. There are still uncertainties regarding the fundamental knowledge of HBOC among doctors specializing in breast cancer, ovarian cancer, and clinical genetics. This encompasses uncertainties pertaining to the provision of information on risk reduction through surgical and surveillance methods, the structure of the information delivery system, and the time frame for HBOC intervention. The research group of the Japanese Breast Cancer Society is planning to conduct a questionnaire survey of three distinct groups: (1) individuals carrying the *BRCA1/2* carriers, (2) medical personnel involved in HBOC, and (3) the general public. The objective of this survey is threefold: first, to disseminate knowledge about genetic medicine and establish a foundation for better genetic medicine; second, to identify the current status of genetic medicine and issues facing those who provide and receive medical care; and third, to gain insight into the perceptions and attitudes of the aforementioned groups toward genetic medicine. The findings of the research are forthcoming.

3.7 Conclusion

HBOC care comprises continuous screening, risk reduction surgery, and multidisciplinary comprehensive care. Furthermore, personalized, specialized, and quality care is required for cancer patients, individuals with no prior cancer history, and their families. Furthermore, the number of multigene panel tests has increased as a consequence of technological advances and cost reductions, which has led to a corresponding rise in interest in genetic medicine, including HBOC care. Nevertheless, there remains a discrepancy between the providers of genetic medicine, who offer services such as surveillance, medical intervention for risk-reducing surgery, and genetic counseling, and those who receive genetic medicine. To address this issue, it is prudent to strengthen the educational infrastructure and develop a skilled workforce for the administration of genetic medicine. In addition to integrating multiple regional medical institutions with the objective of optimizing the utilization of existing medical resources, the implementation of medical telemedicine, including online systems capable of providing treatment for individuals residing beyond the reach of conventional medical facilities, will also prove invaluable.

However, psychological burden is another factor that cannot be overlooked. It can be stated that medical staff who are not engaged in the field of genetic medicine have reported feelings of anxiety during the course of their patients' medical treatment. This suggests the necessity for the implementation of a reinforcement mechanism. Moreover, the domain of genetic medicine encompasses a multitude of decisions, including the determination of the optimal timing for genetic testing, the designation of the appropriate moment to disseminate test results to family members, and the selection between risk-reducing surgery and surveillance. While the concept of "choice" affords clients or *BRCA1/2* carriers a sense of autonomy, it can also become a burdensome responsibility in certain circumstances. It is incumbent upon medical professionals to ensure that they comprehend and align themselves with the values and intentions of the patient in question, and to be mindful of the principles of ShareSDM, which serve to facilitate the formation of a consensus. It is therefore beneficial for psychologists to participate in the genetic counseling phase and in instances where SDM is required, to provide psychological assistance to clients and their families. To this end, it is essential to give priority to the development of human resources and the establishment of systems. It is also important to disseminate correct information about genetic medicine to the general public in order to promote genetic medicine smoothly. Furthermore, it is essential to strive toward the establishment of an equitable healthcare provision system for *BRCA1/2* carriers, and a society in which they can live with peace of mind on an equal footing.

References

1. Nakama M, Matsuyama Y, Murase S, Asano Y, Futamura M, Iinuma K, Ishihara T, Imoto I, Morishige K. A survey of clinical management for HBOC in Japan. J Hereditary Tumors. 2022;22:1–8.
2. Abacan M, Alsubaie L, Barlow-Stewart K, et al. The global state of the genetic counseling profession. Eur J Hum Genet. 2019;27:183–97.
3. Kawai M, Ohtani S, Iwasaki M, et al. The Japanese breast cancer society clinical practice guidelines for epidemiology and prevention of breast cancer, 2022 edition. Breast Cancer. 2024;31:166–78.
4. Kobayashi Y, Masuda K, Hiraswa A, et al. Current status of hereditary breast and ovarian cancer practice among gynecologic oncologists in Japan: a nationwide survey by the Japan Society of Gynecologic Oncology (JSGO). J Gynecol Oncol. 2021;33:e61.
5. George R, Kovak K, Cox SL. Aligning policy to promote cascade genetic screening for prevention and early diagnosis of heritable diseases. J Genet Couns. 2015;24:388–99.
6. Federici G, Soddu S. Variants of uncertain significance in the era of high-throughput genome sequencing: a lesson from breast and ovary cancers. J Exp Clin Cancer Res. 2020;39:46.
7. Fabi A, Cortesi L, Duranti S, et al. Multigenic panels in breast cancer: clinical utility and management of patients with pathogenic variants other than BRCA1/2. Crit Rev Oncol Hematol. 2024;201:104431.
8. McAlarnen L, Stearns K, Uyar D. Challenges of genomic testing for hereditary breast and ovarian cancers. Appl Clin Genet. 2021;14:1–9.
9. Rhiem K, Bücker-Nott H, Hellmich M, et al. Benchmarking of a checklist for the identification of familial risk for breast and ovarian cancers in a prospective cohort. Breast J. 2019;25:455–60.
10. Herold N, Bredow K, Ernst C, et al. Implementing mainstream genetic counseling within the area-wide network of the German consortium hereditary breast and ovarian cancer (GC-HBOC): satisfaction of primary care providers with the provided state-of-the-art training by the Cologne center. J Genet Couns. 2024;33:206–15.
11. Lapointe J, Dorval M, Chiquette J, et al. A collaborative model to implement flexible, accessible and efficient oncogenetic services for hereditary breast and ovarian cancer: the C-MOnGene study. Cancers. 2021;13:2729.
12. Narod SA, Gojska N, Sun P, Tryon A, Kotsopoulos J, Metcalfe K, Akbari MR. The screen project: guided direct-to-consumer genetic testing for breast cancer susceptibility in Canada. Cancers. 2021;13:1894.
13. Aizawa Y, Watanabe A, Kato K. Institutional and social issues surrounding genetic counselors in Japan: current challenges and implications for the global community. Front Genet. 2021;12:646177.
14. Biesecker B. Genetic counseling and the central tenets of practice. Cold Spring Harb Perspect Med. 2020;10:a038968.
15. Ormond KE, Abad PJ, MacLeod R, Nishigaki M, Wessels T-M (2024) The global status of genetic counseling in 2023: What's changed in the past 5 years? Genet Med Open 101887.
16. Kohzaki H. Problems and their solutions in genetic counseling education in Japan. Front Public Heal. 2014;2:100.
17. Meiser B, Woodward P, Gleeson M, et al. Pilot study of an online training program to increase genetic literacy and communication skills in oncology healthcare professionals discussing BRCA1/2 genetic testing with breast and ovarian cancer patients. Fam Cancer. 2022;21:157–66.
18. Berger-Höger B, Vitinius F, Fischer H, et al. Nurse-led decision coaching by specialized nurses for healthy BRCA1/2 gene mutation carriers - adaptation and pilot testing of a curriculum for nurses: a qualitative study. BMC Nurs. 2022;21:42.
19. Isselhard A, Töpper M, Berger-Höger B, et al. Implementation and evaluation of a nurse-led decision-coaching program for healthy breast cancer susceptibility gene (BRCA1/2) mutation carriers: a study protocol for the randomized controlled EDCP-BRCA study. Trials. 2020;21:501.
20. Cook L, Verbrugge J, Schwantes-An T-H, et al. Providing genetic testing and genetic counseling for Parkinson's disease to the community. Genet Med. 2023;25:100907.

Chapter 4
CRRM or Surveillance: An Evidence-Based Individual Decision-Making

Kazunori Kubota

Abstract This chapter explores the management of contralateral breast cancer in patients with *BRCA1* and *BRCA2* mutations, focusing on two primary strategies: contralateral risk-reducing mastectomy (CRRM) and intensified surveillance using imaging techniques such as contrast-enhanced breast MRI. *BRCA* mutation carriers face a significant risk of developing contralateral breast cancer. CRRM significantly reduces the risk of contralateral breast cancer, but the procedure carries surgical risks and potential impacts on quality of life. Surveillance aims to detect cancer early through regular imaging, balancing the psychological burden of ongoing cancer risk with the avoidance of surgical intervention. This document explores the benefits, risks, and implications of each strategy and highlights the importance of making evidence-based, individualized decision-making. The analysis is based on the Japanese Organization of Hereditary Breast and Ovarian Cancer (JOHBOC) guidelines from Japan and recent research findings, aiming to provide comprehensive recommendations for high-risk women.

Keywords *BRCA1/2* · Mastectomy · Surveillance · HBOC · Breast MRI

4.1 Introduction

In the management of hereditary breast cancer, particularly among *BRCA1* and *BRCA2* mutation carriers, the risk of developing contralateral breast cancer is a significant concern. The risk of developing contralateral breast cancer has been reported to be 40% for *BRCA1* and 26% for *BRCA2* by 20 years after the diagnosis of breast cancer [1]. The strategies to manage this risk are critical for improving patient outcomes and quality of life. Two primary strategies have emerged: contralateral

K. Kubota (✉)
Department of Radiology, Dokkyo Medical University Saitama Medical Center, Saitama, Japan
e-mail: kubotard@dokkyomed.ac.jp

A. Sakurai et al. (eds.), *Practical Guide to Hereditary Breast and Ovarian Cancer II*, https://doi.org/10.1007/978-981-96-4329-5_4

risk-reducing mastectomy (CRRM) and intensified surveillance. This chapter explores these strategies in depth, examining their benefits, risks, and implications for patients.

CRRM involves the prophylactic removal of the non-affected breast to prevent the occurrence of contralateral breast cancer, offering a substantial reduction in risk. Surveillance, on the other hand, relies on mainly periodic imaging examinations by contrast-enhanced breast MRI to detect any new malignancies early, allowing for timely intervention. Both approaches have their merits and challenges, and the choice between them is often complex, involving not just medical considerations but also psychological, social, and personal factors.

Based on the Japanese Organization of Hereditary Breast and Ovarian Cancer (JOHBOC) guidelines from Japan [2] and findings from recent studies, this document provides a comprehensive overview of the options available to high-risk women. The process of evidence-based decision-making is important, and for each individual patient, the decision on the course of treatment must be further informed by the patient's own background and perspective as a patient with the disease.

4.2 CRRM: Contralateral Risk-Reducing Mastectomy

4.2.1 Definition and Purpose

CRRM is a surgical intervention aimed at significantly reducing the risk of developing contralateral breast cancer in women who are at high risk due to genetic mutations, particularly *BRCA1* and *BRCA2*, or a strong family history of breast cancer. The procedure involves the removal of the contralateral breast—i.e., the breast that has not been affected by cancer—to prevent the development of a new primary tumor in that breast.

The JOHBOC guidelines [2] present the following clinical question:

CQ1. Is contralateral risk-reducing mastectomy (CRRM) recommended for breast cancer patients with *BRCA* pathogenic variants?

Recommendation. CRRM is conditionally recommended for breast cancer patients with *BRCA* pathogenic variants.

Certainty of evidence "Medium"/Type of recommendation "Conditional recommendation for the intervention in question"/Agreement rate "100% (12/12)"

4.2.2 Indications for CRRM

CRRM is generally considered for women who have already been diagnosed with breast cancer and are found to be at high risk for developing contralateral breast cancer. CRRM may be particularly indicated for women with *BRCA1/2* mutations. The decision to undergo CRRM should be based on a thorough assessment of the patient's risk factors, including age, characteristics of the primary tumor, and presence of other genetic mutations that may elevate the risk of contralateral breast cancer.

In Japan, *BRCA* genetic testing is currently recommended [2] and covered by insurance for the following patients:

- Breast cancer with onset at age 45 years or younger.
- Breast cancer with onset at age 60 or younger and triple-negative subtype.
- Two or more primary breast cancers on both sides or one side.
- Male breast cancer.
- Ovarian, fallopian tube, or peritoneal cancer at the time of breast cancer diagnosis.
- Family history of breast, ovarian, or pancreatic cancer in blood relatives (third-degree relatives).

The National Comprehensive Cancer Network (NCCN) guidelines describe the cumulative risk of developing contralateral breast cancer by age as follows [1, 3, 4]:

In *BRCA1*

20-year cumulative risk: 30%–40%
15-year cumulative risk in premenopausal women: >20%

In *BRCA2*

20-year cumulative risk: 25%
15-year cumulative risk in premenopausal women: >20%

Women under the age of 40 are often considered strong candidates for CRRM, as they face a higher lifetime risk of contralateral breast cancer. Additionally, women with a strong family history of breast cancer or those who have had breast cancer at an early age are also prime candidates for this procedure. Genetic counseling is an important component of the decision-making process, as it helps to clarify the individual's risk and guide the choice between CRRM and other management strategies.

4.2.3 Benefits of CRRM

The most significant benefit of CRRM is the dramatic reduction in the risk of contralateral breast cancer. The JOHBOC guidelines conducted a meta-analysis based on four articles [5–8], and the results showed a significant reduction in the risk of developing contralateral breast cancer with a risk ratio of 0.07 (95% CI: 0.02–0.23, $P < 0.00001$) (Fig. 4.1).

Although it should be noted that the analysis was performed without adjustment for possible publication bias and for the risk reducing salpingo–oophorectomy (RRSO), it is almost certain that CRRM minimizes the risk of developing breast cancer.

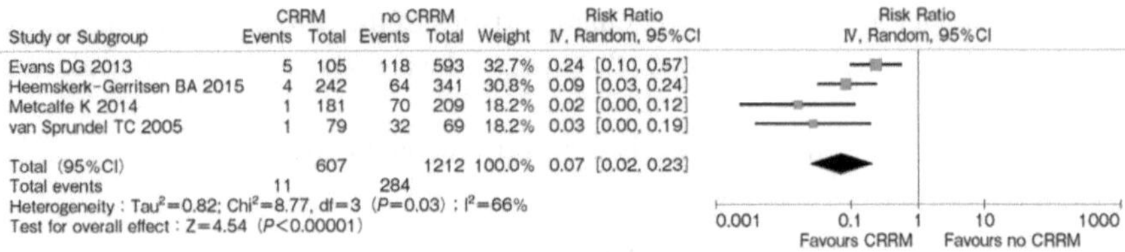

Fig. 4.1 Meta-analysis of contralateral breast risk reduction with CRRM in previously diagnosed breast cancer patients with BRCA pathogenic variants [5–8]

CRRM also has the potential to improve overall survival, particularly in women with *BRCA1/2* mutations. The meta-analysis showed a significant reduction in mortality with HR [HR 0.48 (95% CI 0.35–0.64)], but the issue remains that the effect of RRSO as a confounding factor cannot be completely excluded [1, 4–6].

While the evidence is mixed, some studies suggest that CRRM may confer a modest survival benefit. This potential survival benefit, combined with the reduction in contralateral breast cancer risk, makes CRRM an attractive option for many high-risk women.

Additionally, CRRM may alleviate the psychological burden associated with the fear of developing another breast cancer. For many women, the knowledge that they have significantly reduced their risk of contralateral breast cancer can provide a sense of control and relief from the anxiety that often accompanies the diagnosis of a hereditary cancer syndrome.

4.2.4 Risks and Complications of CRRM

Despite its benefits, CRRM is not without risks. As with any major surgery, there are inherent risks associated with the procedure, including infection, bleeding, and complications related to anesthesia. The risk of surgical complications is heightened in women who undergo simultaneous reconstruction, which is often performed to address the cosmetic and psychological impacts of mastectomy.

Moreover, CRRM can have significant effects on body image and sexual function, as the removal of the breast can lead to feelings of loss and altered self-perception. These effects can be particularly pronounced in younger women, who may place a higher value on their physical appearance and sexual identity. The psychological impact of CRRM should not be underestimated, and patients should be fully informed about the potential consequences of the surgery.

Long-term complications of CRRM can include chronic pain, numbness, and issues related to breast reconstruction. For some women, the physical and psychological challenges associated with CRRM may outweigh the benefits, leading to regret or dissatisfaction with the decision to undergo the procedure. Also, it is not easy to formulate a certain view on the balance between costs and resources.

4.2.5 Recommendation

According to current guidelines, CRRM is conditionally recommended for breast cancer patients with *BRCA* pathogenic variants. However, there is much uncertainty regarding the effect of CRRM on survival because of the influence of RRSO. Also, it is important to note that this recommendation is not a comparison of CRRM with surveillance.

4.3 Surveillance in High-Risk Populations

4.3.1 Definition and Purpose

Surveillance is a nonsurgical approach to managing the risk of contralateral breast cancer that involves regular monitoring of the breast tissue to detect any new malignancies early. This strategy is based on the principle that early detection of breast cancer leads to better outcomes, including improved survival and reduced morbidity.

For women at general risk, the term "screening" is used, which aims to efficiently detect breast cancer in the population. For high-risk groups, the term "surveillance" is used, to detect early-stage breast cancer that can be treated as minimally invasively as possible. Mammography, which has been proven to improve life expectancy, is used to screen for general-risk breast cancer. On the other hand, many breast cancers cannot be detected by mammography alone, especially in dense breasts, which are known to have decreased detection efficiency. In addition, it is now known that some breast cancers can be missed even in the absence of dense breasts, and ultrasound is used in conjunction with mammography in screening [9]. It is known that more breast cancers can be detected by contrast-enhanced breast MRI than by mammography and ultrasound combined [10], and breast MRI is preferred in surveillance for high-risk groups.

For women at high risk of contralateral breast cancer, particularly those with *BRCA1/2* mutations, surveillance is an important component of their overall management plan.

4.3.2 Guidelines for Surveillance

The JOHBOC guidelines [2] state the following in the Clinical Question

CQ4. Is surveillance with contrast-enhanced breast MRI recommended for the preserved and contralateral breast of breast cancer patients with *BRCA* pathogenic variants?

Recommendation. Surveillance with contrast-enhanced breast MRI is conditionally recommended for the preserved and contralateral breast of breast cancer patients with *BRCA* pathogenic variants.

Certainty of Evidence "Weak"/Type of Recommendation "Conditional recommendation for such intervention"/Agreement Rate "100% (13/13)".

Surveillance of breast cancer using contrast-enhanced breast MRI in *BRCA* pathogenic variant carriers has been shown to increase sensitivity without decreasing specificity. However, surveillance of breast cancer using contrast-enhanced breast MRI in *BRCA* pathogenic variant carriers who have not yet developed breast or ovarian cancer is currently not covered by insurance in Japan, and patients who wish to undergo this service must pay for it themselves. It is recommended that the surveillance be conducted at a medical institution that has specialists with sufficient knowledge of contrast-enhanced breast MRI, has a good collaboration with facilities that can perform MRI-guided biopsies, and has a system for genetic counseling and follow-up after the screening.

4.3.3 Benefits of Surveillance

The benefit of surveillance is the ability to detect cancer at an early stage, when it is most treatable. In a qualitative systematic review of 11 observational studies [10–20], the sensitivity of breast cancer detection in surveillance that included MRI (66.7–100%) was higher than in surveillance that did not include MRI (19–81%).

Regarding the false positive rate, a qualitative systematic review of nine observational studies [10–18] showed that the false positive rate for surveillance including MRI was 45% in only one study and less than 10% in the others.

Early detection of breast cancer is associated with improved outcomes, including higher survival rates and less aggressive treatment options. A qualitative systematic review of three observational studies [21–23] showed higher survival rates for surveillance that included MRI than for surveillance that did not include MRI (95.3% vs. 87.7% and 100% vs. 85.5% for 10-year and 3-year survival rates, respectively;100% vs. 92%). For women who are closely monitored, the likelihood of detecting a new tumor before it becomes advanced is high, which can lead to better overall outcomes.

Another advantage of surveillance is that it allows women to avoid the risks and complications associated with surgery. For women who are not ready or willing to undergo CRRM, surveillance offers a viable alternative that allows them to preserve their breasts while still managing their risk of contralateral breast cancer.

4.3.4 Risks and Limitations of Surveillance

While surveillance is less invasive than CRRM, it is not without its risks and limitations. One of the primary challenges of surveillance is the potential for false positives, which can lead to unnecessary biopsies, anxiety, and even surgery. False positives are particularly common in younger women, whose dense breast tissue can make it difficult to distinguish between benign and malignant lesions.

Moreover, surveillance does not prevent the occurrence of contralateral breast cancer, but rather aims to detect it early. This means that women who choose surveillance must live with the ongoing risk of developing another breast cancer, which can be a significant psychological burden. The need for regular imaging and clinical examinations can also be stressful, particularly for women who experience anxiety related to medical procedures.

Another limitation of surveillance is the possibility that cancer will be detected at a more advanced stage, despite regular monitoring. While surveillance aims to catch cancer early, there is always a risk that a new tumor will develop and progress before it is detected. This risk is higher in women who have dense breast tissue or other factors that make it difficult to detect cancer on imaging.

Finally, the long-term impact of radiation exposure from regular mammography is a concern, particularly for younger women. While the risk of radiation-induced cancer is generally low, it is still a consideration for women who begin surveillance at a young age and are exposed to radiation over many years.

4.3.5 Surveillance Methods

The National Comprehensive Cancer Network (NCCN) guidelines [3] recommend the following examinations for individuals with *BRCA* pathogenic variants or a family history of breast cancer with a lifetime risk of >20% for the development of breast cancer.

- Breast awareness starting at age 18 years.
- Clinical breast examination, every 6–12 months, starting at age 25 years.
- Breast screening.

Age 25–29 years, annual breast MRI screening with and without contrast (or mammogram, only if MRI is unavailable) or individualized based on family history if a breast cancer diagnosis before age 30 is present.

Age 30–75 years, annual mammogram and breast MRI screening with and without contrast.

Age > 75 years, management should be considered on an individual basis.

The ESMO (European Society for Medical Oncology) guidelines [24] recommend annual contrast-enhanced breast MRI for HBOC patients starting 5 years before the youngest affected family member or by age 30 at the latest. However, if MRI every 6 months is not feasible, ultrasound or mammography can be used to compensate.

In the realm of surveillance, new imaging technologies are being developed to improve the accuracy and effectiveness of breast cancer screening. Digital breast tomosynthesis (DBT), also known as 3D mammography, is one such technology that has shown promise in improving the detection of breast cancer, particularly in women with dense breast tissue. DBT provides a more detailed, three-dimensional view of the breast, which can help reduce the number of false positives and improve the detection of small tumors.

In breast ultrasound, the diagnostic performance of handheld ultrasound systems depends on the skill of the operator. Recently, an automated breast ultrasound scanner (ABUS), which scans the entire breast automatically has been introduced. However, there is still little evidence regarding its ability to detect breast cancer in HBOC surveillance. On the other hand, since ultrasound is a noninvasive and repeatable examination method, it may be useful to perform ultrasound examinations at half the interval of MRI surveillance (e.g., every 6 months for ultrasound compared with every year for MRI), for short-term follow-up of significant findings that require follow-up, and for those who cannot undergo MRI. The role of ultrasound in HBOC surveillance is a subject for future research.

Another emerging area of research is the use of artificial intelligence (AI) and machine learning to analyze imaging data. AI has the potential to improve the accuracy of breast cancer screening by identifying patterns that may be missed by human radiologists. Early studies suggest that AI-assisted imaging analysis could reduce the number of false positives and negatives, leading to more accurate and reliable surveillance.

4.4 Comparison of CRRM and Surveillance

4.4.1 Efficacy in Risk Reduction

When considering the efficacy of CRRM and surveillance, the most crucial factor is the degree of risk reduction each strategy provides. CRRM offers the most significant reduction in the risk of developing contralateral breast cancer, with studies indicating a reduction ratio of 0.07. This is a substantial reduction, and for many women, it represents a definitive strategy for managing their cancer risk.

In contrast, surveillance does not reduce the risk of developing contralateral breast cancer but rather focuses on early detection. The success of surveillance hinges on the timely and accurate identification of cancerous changes, which can then be treated before the disease progresses. While this strategy can be effective in catching cancers early, it inherently carries a greater risk of missing a cancer or detecting it at a more advanced stage. This is particularly concerning for younger women, whose dense breast tissue can make it more difficult to detect abnormalities through imaging alone.

Because of the risk of developing ovarian cancer in *BRCA* pathogenic variant carriers and the current lack of effective prevention or surveillance methods for ovarian cancer, RRSO is recommended. The effect of ovarian removal on improved survival must also be considered; few studies have evaluated CRRM overall survival after adjusting for RRSO confounders, so the effect of RRSO may have a higher impact.

Depending on the stage and subtype of breast cancer that has developed, additional drug therapy will be required, and the extent to which this is effective in reducing breast cancer incidence and mortality will also be an issue. There may be cases in which CRRM is not highly effective in patients with advanced stages of breast cancer who are at risk of metastasis or recurrence. If the postoperative recurrence-free period is long, the effectiveness of CRRM may be reevaluated. In addition, in imaging surveillance, it is important to know how well contrast-enhanced breast MRI can be performed and whether MRI-detected lesions can be approached appropriately. There are also significant issues such as what should be done for patients who are unable to undergo MRI.

The psychological impact of surgical breast loss and the relief of reduced risk of disease are different for each patient. It may also change over time. It is also likely that individual patients will differ in their perceptions of the respective benefit and harm outcomes of CRRM and surveillance.

The decision-making process should involve a comprehensive discussion between the patient and her healthcare provider, including an assessment of her individual risk factors, preferences, and psychological readiness for surgery. Shared decision-making tools and genetic counseling can be valuable resources in this process, helping to ensure that the patient makes an informed choice that aligns with her values and goals.

4.4.2 Case Study

A woman in her 40s with no family history was found to have a 13 mm mass in her left breast by an ultrasound screening and was diagnosed with triple-negative breast cancer following a core-needle biopsy. Contrast-enhanced breast MRI revealed a localized mass (arrow head) in the left breast. There was no evidence of multiple lesions besides biopsy-confirmed fibroadenoma (arrow), and there were no abnormal findings in the right breast (Fig. 4.2). The clinical staging was determined as T1cN0M0, stage IA. *BRCA1* mutation was detected by genetic testing, and after consulting with the patient regarding treatment options, it was decided to proceed

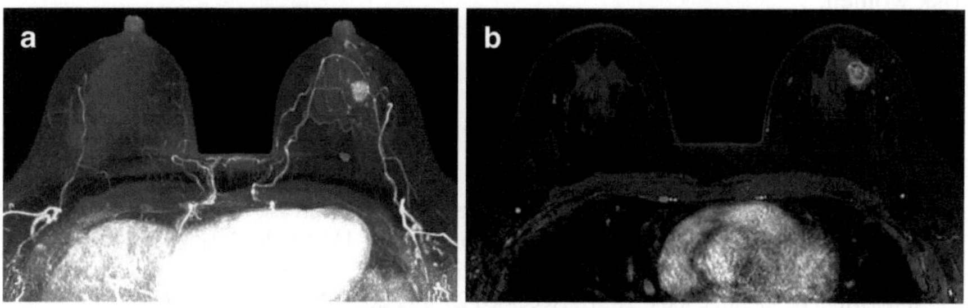

Fig. 4.2 Contrast-enhanced breast MRI. (**a**) MIP image, (**b**) axial image

with a mastectomy of the affected breast, contralateral risk-reducing mastectomy (CRRM), and risk-reducing salpingo-oophorectomy (RRSO) after neoadjuvant chemotherapy.

Although breast-conserving therapy for the affected side and subsequent surveillance was also considered, the detection of the *BRCA* mutation broadened the scope of treatment options to include surgery and pharmacological interventions for the contralateral breast and ovaries.

This scenario highlights the importance of personalized care and the need for tailored recommendations based on the individual patient's circumstances and preferences.

4.4.3 Considerations

The management of contralateral breast cancer risk in high-risk women is a complex task that requires careful consideration of various factors, including the risk of contralateral breast cancer, the impact on survival, the psychological and physical effects, and the patient's values and preferences. While CRRM offers the most significant reduction in contralateral breast cancer risk, it comes with its own set of challenges, including surgical risks and potential impacts on quality of life. Surveillance, while less invasive, requires a lifelong commitment to regular monitoring and carries its psychological burden.

The decision between CRRM and surveillance should be made collaboratively, with the patient fully informed and actively involved in the process. Healthcare providers must offer comprehensive counseling, considering the latest evidence-based guidelines, emerging research, and the individual patient's circumstances. Ultimately, the goal is to provide personalized care that aligns with the patient's values and goals, ensuring that she feels confident and supported in her decision.

As research continues to evolve, the strategies for managing contralateral breast cancer risk will likely become more refined, with new tools and technologies enhancing both CRRM and surveillance options. The ongoing commitment to personalized medicine and ethical care will be essential in guiding patients through these complex decisions, helping to improve outcomes and quality of life for high-risk women.

References

1. Kuchenbaecker KB, Hopper JL, Barnes DR, et al. Risks of breast, ovarian, and contralateral breast cancer for BRCA1 and BRCA2 mutation carriers. JAMA. 2017;317(23):2402–16.
2. Guidelines for Diagnosis and Treatment of Hereditary Breast and Ovarian Cancer 2021. https://johboc.jp/guidebook_2021/. Accessed 25 Aug 2024.
3. NCCN clinical practice guidelines in oncology. Genetic/familial high risk assessment:breast, ovarian and pancreatic. Version 3. 2024.

4. Yadav S, Boddicker NJ, Na J, et al. Contralateral breast cancer risk among carriers of germline pathogenic variants in ATM, BRCA1, BRCA2, CHEK2, and PALB2. J Clin Oncol. 2023;41:1703–13.
5. Evans DG, Ingham SL, Baildam A, et al. Contralateral mastectomy improves survival in women with BRCA1/2—associated breast cancer. Breast Cancer Res Treat. 2013;140(1):135–42.
6. Heemskerk-Gerritsen BAM, Rookus MA, Aalfs CM, Ausems MGEM, Collée JM, Jansen L, Kets C, Keymeulen KBMI, Koppert LB, MeijersHeijboer HEJ, Mooij TM, Tollenaar RAEM, Vasen HFA, HEBON, Hooning MJ, Seynaeve C. Improved overall survival after contralateral risk—reducing mastectomy in BRCA1/2 mutation carriers with a history of unilateral breast cancer:a prospective analysis. Int J Cancer. 2015;136(3):668–77.
7. Metcalfe K, Gershman S, Ghadirian P, et al. Contralateral mastectomy and survival after breast cancer in carriers of BRCA1 and BRCA2 mutations:retrospective analysis. BMJ. 2014;348:g226.
8. van Sprundel TC, Schmidt MK, Rookus MA, et al. Risk reduction of contralateral breast cancer and survival after contralateral prophylactic mastectomy in BRCA1 or BRCA2 mutation carriers. Br J Cancer. 2005;93(3):287–92.
9. Ohuchi N, Suzuki A, Sobue T, Kawai M, Yamamoto S, Zheng YF, et al; J-START investigator groups. Sensitivity and specificity of mammography and adjunctive ultrasonography to screen for breast cancer in the Japan strategic anti-cancer randomized trial(J-START): a randomised controlled trial. Lancet 2016; 387(10016): 341-8.me
10. Kuhl CK, Schrading S, Leutner CC, et al. Mammography, breast ultrasound, and magnetic resonance imaging for surveillance of women at high familial risk for breast cancer. J Clin Oncol. 2005;23(33):8469–76.
11. Guindalini RSC, Zheng Y, Abe H, et al. Intensive surveillance with biannual dynamic contrastenhanced magnetic resonance imaging downstages breast cancer in BRCA1 mutation carriers. Clin Cancer Res. 2019;25(6):1786–94.
12. Riedl CC, Luft N, Bernhart C, et al. Triple-modality screening trial for familial breast cancer underlines the importance of magnetic resonance imaging and questions the role of mammography and ultrasound regardless of patient mutation status, age, and breast density. J Clin Oncol. 2015;33(10):1128–35.
13. Warner E, Plewes DB, Hill KA, et al. Surveillance of BRCA1 and BRCA2 mutation carriers with magnetic resonance imaging, ultrasound, mammography, and clinical breast examination. JAMA. 2004;292(11):1317–25.
14. Bosse K, Graeser M, Goßmann A, et al. Supplemental screening ultrasound increases cancer detection yield in BRCA1 and BRCA2 mutation carriers. Arch Gynecol Obstet. 2014;289(3):663–70.
15. Kriege M, Brekelmans CT, Obdeijn IM, et al. Factors affecting sensitivity and specificity of screening mammography and MRI in women with an inherited risk for breast cancer. Breast Cancer Res Treat. 2006;100(1):109–19.
16. Passaperuma K, Warner E, Causer PA, et al. Long-term results of screening with magnetic resonance imaging in women with BRCA mutations. Br J Cancer. 2012;107(1):24–30.
17. Rijnsburger AJ, Obdeijn IM, Kaas R, et al. BRCA1-associated breast cancers present differently from BRCA2-associated and familial cases:long-term follow-up of the Dutch MRISC screening study. J Clin Oncol. 2010;28(36):5265–73.
18. Bick U, Engel C, Krug B, et al. German consortium for hereditary breast and ovarian cancer(GCHBOC). High-risk breast cancer surveillance with MRI:10-year experience from the German consortium for hereditary breast and ovarian cancer. Breast Cancer Res Treat. 2019;175(1):217–28.
19. Cortesi L, Canossi B, Battista R, et al. Breast ultrasonography(BU)in the screening protocol for women at hereditary-familial risk of breast cancer:has the time come to rethink the role of BU according to different risk categories? Int J Cancer. 2019;144(5):1001–9.
20. Hagen AI, Kvistad KA, Maehle L, et al. Sensitivity of MRI versus conventional screening in the diagnosis of BRCA-associated breast cancer in a national prospective series. Breast. 2007;16(4):367–74.

21. Evans DG, Kesavan N, Lim Y, et al. MRI breast screening in high-risk women:cancer detection and survival analysis. Breast Cancer Res Treat. 2014;145(3):663–72.
22. Chéreau E, Uzan C, Balleyguier C, et al. Characteristics, treatment, and outcome of breast cancers diagnosed in BRCA1 and BRCA2 gene mutation carriers in intensive screening programs including magnetic resonance imaging. Clin Breast Cancer. 2010;10(2):113–8.
23. Evans DG, Harkness EF, Howell A, et al. Intensive breast screening in BRCA2 mutation carriers is associated with reduced breast cancer specific and all cause mortality. Hered Cancer Clin Pract. 2016;14:8.
24. Sessa C, Balmaña J, Bober SL, et al. ESMO guidelines committee. Electronic address: clinicalguidelines@esmo.org. Risk reduction and screening of cancer in hereditary breast-ovarian cancer syndromes: ESMO clinical practice guideline. Ann Oncol. 2023;34(1):33–47.

Chapter 5
RRSO for Aged Patients with Breast Cancer

Masayuki Sekine, Rie Nakamura, Tomoko Nakamoto, Yukiko Chinen, Yoshino Kinjo, Natsuki Tamashiro, Yuko Shimoji, Yusuke Taira, Yoshihisa Arakaki, Takuma Oyama, and Wataru Kudaka

Abstract In Japan, risk-reducing salpingo-oophorectomy (RRSO), which is now covered by insurance, is rapidly increasing for breast cancer patients with *BRCA1/2* germline mutation. In this chapter, we first review new findings from recent clinical trials on RRSO for the prevention of breast, ovarian, fallopian tube, and peritoneal cancers. Next, we discuss measures to address recent issues in clinical practice regarding the preventive treatment of secondary cancers in breast cancer patients, especially in elderly patients. Specifically, these are the following questions. (1) Should RRSO be aggressively performed on breast cancer patients? (2) Does RRSO reduce the risk of breast cancer recurrence and the risk of developing secondary breast cancer? (3) Do anticancer drugs used in the treatment of breast cancer decrease the risk of developing ovarian cancer? Finally, the results of the analysis of the Japan Organization of Hereditary Breast and Ovarian Cancer (JOHBOC) national registry will be presented, detailing the differences in cancer risk by gene, particularly in age at onset. Based on the data, we discuss how information on risk-reducing surgery should be provided in genetic counseling for breast cancer patients.

Keywords Risk-reducing salpingo-oophorectomy (RRSO) · *BRCA1* · *BRCA2* · Ovarian cancer · Breast cancer

5.1 Introduction

In Japan, preventive care for breast and/or ovarian cancer patients with a germline mutation in *BRCA1/2* gene (g*BRCA1/2*m) who may develop breast and/or ovarian cancer in the future was covered by insurance in April 2020. The items covered in

M. Sekine (✉) · R. Nakamura · T. Nakamoto · Y. Chinen · Y. Kinjo · N. Tamashiro
Y. Shimoji · Y. Taira · Y. Arakaki · T. Oyama · W. Kudaka
Department of Obstetrics and Gynecology, Graduate School of Medical Science, University of the Ryukyus, Okinawa, Japan
e-mail: msekine@med.u-ryukyu.ac.jp; https://researchmap.jp/masa88

A. Sakurai et al. (eds.), *Practical Guide to Hereditary Breast and Ovarian Cancer II*, https://doi.org/10.1007/978-981-96-4329-5_5

this preventive care include (1) *BRCA* genetic testing and genetic counseling, (2) risk-reducing salpingo-oophorectomy (RRSO), contralateral risk-reducing mastectomy (CRRM), and breast reconstruction for breast cancer patients with g*BRCA1/2*m, (3) bilateral risk-reducing mastectomy (BRRM) and breast reconstruction for ovarian cancer patients with g*BRCA1/2*m, (4) breast cancer surveillance and/or ovarian cancer surveillance for breast and/or ovarian cancer patients with g*BRCA1/2*m.

In this chapter, we would like to discuss the latest topics on RRSO for breast cancer patients, especially for elderly patients, as well as the data from the analysis of a gradually increasing number of Japanese patients with hereditary breast and ovarian cancer (HBOC).

5.2 Problems with RRSO for Aged Patients with Breast Cancer

Until now, genetic testing for cancer susceptibility genes, such as *BRCA1/2* gene, has been performed on "families with many cancer-affected individuals." Recent advances in cancer genomic medicine have led to the rapid spread of *BRCA* genetic testing, as more cancer patients undergo multigene panel testing as well as companion diagnosis for poly(ADP-ribose) polymerase (PARP) inhibitors. As a result, many patients with g*BRCA1/2*m have been found, and genetic counseling on surveillance and risk-reducing surgery for family members is rapidly increasing [1].

For breast cancer patients, the number of patients undergoing *BRCA* genetic testing has increased dramatically for the purposes of (1) surgical procedure selection, (2) companion diagnosis of PARP inhibitors, and (3) health management of family members. In addition, *BRCA* genetic testing may be useful in predicting sensitivity to cytotoxic anticancer agents involved in homologous recombination repair, such as platinum drugs.

In this context, the following issues have been raised in clinical practice regarding RRSO for aged patients with breast cancer:

1. Should patients be actively encouraged to undergo RRSO for ovarian cancer that they may develop in the future after careful consideration of the prognosis for breast cancer?
2. Can RRSO reduce the risk of breast cancer recurrence and development of secondary breast cancer?
3. Can we expect to reduce the risk of developing ovarian cancer with drugs used for breast cancer?
4. Are there any unique Japanese data on the risk reduction effect of RRSO?

It is difficult to make a generalized statement because each breast cancer patient has a different condition, treatment, and attitude toward preventive medicine; however, we will explain what has become clear from the data accumulated so far.

5.3 Risk Reduction Effect on Ovarian and Breast Cancer

Three meta-analyses of the effect of RRSO in reducing the risk of ovarian and breast cancer were reported by Rebbeck et al. [2], Marchetti et al. [3] and Eleje et al. [4] They found a 79–94% risk reduction effect for ovarian cancer and a 42–51% risk reduction effect for breast cancer. It is expected that premenopausal women who undergo oophorectomy will have a reduced risk of developing breast cancer, an estrogen-dependent tumor. However, since a high proportion of breast cancer patients with g*BRCA1*m have estrogen-independent triple-negative breast cancer, a mechanism of action other than a reduction in estrogen levels is speculated as a mechanism of breast cancer risk reduction.

Wang et al. reported in a meta-analysis that a risk reduction effect for breast cancer was observed for both *BRCA1/2*g *BRCA1*m and g*BRCA2*m [*BRCA1*: HR = 0.63 (95% CI: 0.49–0.81), *BRCA2*: HR = 0.51 (95% CI: 0.34–0.75)] in 2022 [5]. Regarding the difference in risk reduction effect by time since RRSO, a reduction in breast cancer risk was observed for both g*BRCA1*m and g*BRCA2*m less than 5 years after RRSO [*BRCA1*: HR = 0.60 (95% CI: 0.40–0.89), *BRCA2*: HR = 0.42 (95% CI: 0.20–0.86)]. On the other hand, there was no reduction in the risk of breast cancer by RRSO for either g*BRCA1* or g*BRCA2*m more than 5 years after RRSO. In a meta-analysis at 2023, Gaba et al. reported that there was no risk reduction in either primary or contralateral breast cancer risk for g*BRCA1/2*m overall, in contrast to a reduction in breast cancer-specific mortality [RR: 0.26 (95% CI: 0.18–0.39)] [6]. In a subgroup analysis, there was no reduction in breast cancer risk in g*BRCA1*m. However, there was a reduction in breast cancer risk in g*BRCA2*m [RR: 0.63 (95%CI: 0.41–0.97)]. Conclusions regarding the effect of RRSO on the risk of breast cancer are inconsistent.

The following questions were raised regarding the age at which patients should undergo RRSO. The question is whether premenopausal RRSO counteract the reduction in breast and ovarian cancer because of the increase in hyperlipidemia-induced "stroke" and "myocardial infarction" that occurs with premature menopause. A prospective cohort study by Domchek et al. provides an answer to this question [7]. In a study of 2482 women with g*BRCA1/2*m, 40% of the subjects received RRSO. In the group that received RRSO, there was a significant 56% reduction in breast cancer-specific mortality, a significant 79% reduction in ovarian cancer-specific mortality, and a significant 60% reduction in all-cause mortality. When the age at which patients received RRSO was analyzed separately for "<50 years" and ">50 years," HR = 0.41 for the "<50 years" group and HR = 0.37 for the ">50 years" group, indicating that there was no difference in risk reduction in all-cause mortality.

Wang et al. analyzed the difference in the risk-reducing effect of RRSO on breast cancer between "<50 years" and ">50 years" in a meta-analysis [5]. In the "<50 years" group, both g*BRCA1*m and g*BRCA2*m showed a significant risk reduction of breast cancer by RRSO [*BRCA1*: HR = 0.48 (95% CI: 0.30–0.77), *BRCA2*: HR = 0.22 (95% CI: 0.08–0.65)]. However, in the ">50 years" group, no risk reduction effect for breast cancer was observed for both g*BRCA1*m and g*BRCA2*m. Although several studies suggest a benefit of RRSO for breast cancer risk reduction, it remains unclear to what extent "differences in the timing of RRSO" affect the effect [8, 9].

The reduced risk of all-cause mortality and prolonged overall survival (OS) attributable to RRSO have also been analyzed in two meta-analyses by Marchetti et al. [3] and Eleje et al. [4] after the prospective cohort study by Domchek et al. [7] As a result, both meta-analyses reported a significant risk reduction effect of 68%. In a recent meta-analysis, Xiao et al. examined g*BRCA1/2*m divided into breast cancer-naïve and previously diagnosed and found a prolonged OS effect in both groups [HR: 0.27 (95% CI: 0.10–0.43), HR: 0.33 (95% CI: 0.28–0.38)] in 2019 [10].

5.4 Occult Cancer Detection and Surveillance for Peritoneal Cancer

The detection rate of occult cancer (serous adenocarcinoma at ovary/fallopian tube/peritoneum) found in RRSO was reported to be 1.5% in g*BRCA1*m and 0.6% in g*BRCA2*m [11]. In g*BRCA1*m, the prevalence of ovarian/fallopian tube/peritoneal cancer in RRSO was 1.5% for those younger than 40 years and 3.8% for those 40–49 years, with the highest incidence in the age group 50–59 years (annual risk = 1.7%). On the other hand, the age group with the highest incidence of g*BRCA2*m was 60–69 years (annual risk = 0.6%) [12].

The cumulative risk of being diagnosed with peritoneal cancer after RRSO was 2.5% at 5 years and 3.5% at 10 years for g*BRCA1/2*m; the cumulative risk was 2.8% at 5 years and 3.9% at 10 years for g*BRCA1*m [13]. Harmsen et al. [14] and Finch et al. [15] reported that the time from RRSO to the development of peritoneal cancer is approximately 5 years.

Serous tubal intraepithelial cancer (STIC) can be found in excised fallopian tubes by RRSO. In the absence of STIC, the cumulative incidence of peritoneal cancer was 0.3% at 5 years and 0.9% at 10 years after RRSO. In comparison, the cumulative incidence of peritoneal cancer in patients with STIC was reported to be 10.5% at 5 years and 27.5% at 10 years after RRSO [16]. In a meta-analysis by Zakhour et al., the median time from RRSO to diagnosis of peritoneal cancer in the presence of STIC was 48 months (18–118 months) [17]. The incidence of future development of peritoneal cancer is extremely high in patients with STIC; therefore, such patients should be followed closely. However, as with ovarian cancer, there is no established surveillance for the development of peritoneal cancer.

5.5 Differences in Risk Reduction Effect by Previous Breast Cancer

A study analyzing whether the risk-reducing effect of RRSO on women who have already developed breast cancer is similar to that of women who have not yet developed the disease is the prospective cohort study by Domchek et al. [7] mentioned previously. The risk reduction effect on ovarian cancer and breast cancer was analyzed by classifying the subjects into breast cancer-naïve and breast cancer-previous. They found a significant risk reduction effect for ovarian cancer regardless of whether the patient had developed breast cancer or not, with more risk reduction among those who had previously developed breast cancer. On the other hand, regarding the risk reduction effect of breast cancer, a significant difference was found in women who had not developed breast cancer (HR = 0.54, 95% CI: 0.37–0.79), but not in those who had previously developed breast cancer (HR = 1.00, 95% CI: 0.56–1.77). Furthermore, they reported a 46% reduction in risk of first breast cancer, but no reduction in risk of second breast cancer.

In a prospective cohort study by Heemskerk-Gerritsen et al. using a person-year method to minimize bias, the analysis showed no effect of RRSO on breast cancer risk reduction [18]. The results of a recent meta-analysis by Xiao et al. showed that RRSO reduced the risk of developing breast cancer as well as ovarian cancer and all-cause mortality in both breast cancer-naïve and previously diagnosed patients [10]. The risk of breast cancer was reduced in both breast cancer-naïve and previously diagnosed patients, but the risk reduction effect was greater in previously diagnosed patients. The risk reduction effect on all-cause mortality was similar for both breast cancer-naïve and breast cancer-experienced patients. There is no agreement in the results regarding the effect of RRSO on reducing the risk of breast cancer.

5.6 Differences in Risk Reduction by *BRCA1* and *BRCA2* Genes

Domchek et al. reported a significant risk reduction in all-cause mortality with g*BRCA1*m (HR = 0.38, 95% CI: 0.24–0.62), but not with g*BRCA2*m (HR = 0.52, 95%CI: 0.22–1.23) in a prospective cohort study. Subsequently, Finch et al. also found that RRSO reduced all-cause mortality at all ages in g*BRCA1*m, but in g*BRCA2*m, the mortality reduction was associated only with ages 41–60 years [12].

A meta-analysis by Eleje et al. also reported a reduction in risk of breast cancer with g*BRCA1*m, but not with g*BRCA2*m [4]. In a case series by Choi et al., the risk-reducing effect of breast cancer for g*BRCA1*m persisted over time, whereas g*BRCA2*m showed no risk-reducing effect 5 years or more after RRSO [19]. On the other hand, a meta-analysis by Gaba et al. [6] and a prospective cohort study by Kauff et al. [20] reported no reduction in breast cancer risk with g*BRCA1*m, but with g*BRCA2*m. In addition, a meta-analysis by Xiao et al. found a significant reduction in all-cause mortality and risk of developing breast cancer in both breast cancer-naïve and previously diagnosed patients, as well as in both g*BRCA1*m and g*BRCA2*m [10]. However, the reduction in all-cause mortality in women with g*BRCA2*m was not significant in breast cancer-naïve patients.

As described above, the results are not in agreement regarding the difference in risk-reducing effect of RRSO by *BRCA1* and *BRCA2* genes, however, the following explanation can be given as to why the risk reduction effect of breast cancer differs between g*BRCA1*m and g*BRCA2*m. Okano et al. reported that hormone-sensitive breast cancer accounts for about 17% of Japanese breast cancer patients with g*BRCA1*m, and the so-called triple-negative breast cancer accounts for more than 80% [21]. On the other hand, approximately 80% of breast cancer patients with g*BRCA2*m are hormone sensitive. Therefore, we can speculate that RRSO may contribute significantly to the improvement of breast cancer prognosis in patients with g*BRCA2*m. However, the results of the analysis using real-world data do not necessarily follow the above theory.

5.7 Reducing the Risk of Developing Ovarian Cancer in the Future with Therapeutic Agents for Breast Cancer

The cytotoxic agents frequently used in the treatment of breast cancer include anthracyclines (e.g., doxorubicin, epirubicin), taxanes (e.g., paclitaxel, docetaxel), and alkylating agents (e.g., cyclophosphamide). Combination chemotherapy of anthracyclines (doxorubicin) and alkylating agents (cyclophosphamide) is widely used as first-line treatment for breast cancer. In addition, PARP inhibitors have recently been introduced. PARP inhibitors have been approved for the treatment of metastatic breast cancer patients with g*BRCA1/2*m. PARP inhibitors used for breast cancer patients with g*BRCA1/2*m have been shown to improve overall survival by inhibiting metastasis and recurrence [22].

Anticancer agents that cause DNA double-strand breaks and involve homologous recombination repair may be more sensitive to cancer patients with g*BRCA1/2*m. The most common drugs are PARP inhibitors (e.g., olaparib and niraparib) and platinum-based chemotherapy agents (e.g., cisplatin, carboplatin, and oxaliplatin), which are currently the key drugs in the treatment of ovarian cancer. There is hope that "platinum-based chemotherapy agents" and "PARP inhibitors," which are highly sensitive to ovarian cancer patients, may contribute to reducing the risk of developing ovarian cancer in the future when used as treatment for breast cancer patients with g*BRCA1/2*m. Anthracyclines, topoisomerase inhibitors (e.g., irinotecan, topotecan, etoposide), and alkylating agents are also believed to cause DNA double-strand breaks.

Theoretically, those agents may reduce the risk of developing primary ovarian cancer by inhibiting the growth of microscopic cancer cells in the ovary, although this speculation has not been evaluated as "prevention against ovarian cancer." Currently, there is no evidence that treatment of breast cancer patients with g*BRCA1/2*m using "platinum-based chemotherapy agents" or "PARP inhibitors" reduces the risk of developing ovarian cancer in the future.

5.8 Other Options Besides RRSO to Prevent Ovarian Cancer

In a study of high-risk groups for ovarian cancer, including g*BRCA1/2*m, surveillance was performed by serum CA125 testing based on the risk of ovarian cancer algorithm (ROCA) every 3 or 4 months and transvaginal ultrasonography (every year or when ROCA score increased). The results suggested that this screening algorithm may increase the proportion of cases with early detection of ovarian cancer; however, it remained unclear whether it would reduce ovarian cancer mortality. Some guidelines, such as European Society for Medical Oncology (ESMO), describe CA125 testing and transvaginal ultrasound every 6 months as a method of surveillance, though their recommendations are currently at a low level [23].

Regarding chemoprevention with oral contraceptives (OC), several meta-analyses have shown that oral OC reduce the risk of ovarian cancer by about 50% in women with g*BRCA1/2*m. [24, 25] Furthermore, it has been reported that the risk of ovarian cancer decreases with longer duration of OC use [26]. There is no consensus on whether OC use increases the risk of breast cancer, with some reports showing no change in risk and others showing an increased risk [25].

In conclusion, it is difficult to recommend OC use in patients with breast cancer for the following reasons:

1. OC administration to patients with breast cancer is contraindicated in Japan.
2. Although several meta-analyses have shown a significant reduction in the risk of ovarian cancer, the results of RCT have not yet been presented.
3. Unlike RRSO, no risk reduction of breast cancer is expected.

Furthermore, thrombosis as a side effect is a major concern. There is an interesting report on the administration of hormonal agents as hormone replacement therapy. Hormone replacement therapy tends to reduce the risk of breast cancer in women who receive estrogen alone compared to those who receive estrogen and progesterone combined (OR = 0.62; 95% CI, 0.29–1.31) [8].

5.9 Age of Onset of Ovarian and Breast Cancer in *BRCA* Mutation Carriers in Japan

The National Comprehensive Cancer Network (NCCN) guideline describes that while it is recommended that g*BRCA1*m undergo RRSO at age 35–40 years, an extension of RRSO to age 45 years may be considered for g*BRCA2*m [27]. This description is based on data from Antoniou et al. in a meta-analysis of 22 reports (Table 5.1) [28]. The relative risk of developing breast and ovarian cancer in women with g*BRCA1/2*m in their 20s to 60s is compared with the risk of developing these cancers in the general population. For breast cancer, both g*BRCA1*m and g*BRCA2*m have an increased risk of developing the disease starting in their 20s. On the other hand, for ovarian cancer, the risk of developing the disease increases from the 30s for g*BRCA1*m and from the 40s for g*BRCA2*m. However, this statement is not based on Japanese data. The Japanese have a lower incidence of ovarian cancer and a higher age of onset of ovarian cancer than Western women [29, 30].

In Japan, when risk-reducing surgery was not covered by insurance, the number of women willing to undergo RRSO was extremely low compared to Western countries [31]. In the Japanese national data reported in 2019, the peak age of RRSO was

Table 5.1 Relative risk (95% CI) for cancer development in *BRCA* mutation carriers compared to the general population

	BRCA1		*BRCA2*	
Age	Breast cancer	Ovarian cancer	Breast cancer	Ovarian cancer
20 ~ 29	17 (4.2–71)	1	19 (4.5–81)	1
30 ~ 39	33 (23–49)	49 (21–111)	16 (9.3–29)	1
40 ~ 49	32 (24–43)	68 (42–111)	9.9 (6.1–16)	6.3 (1.4–28)
50 ~ 59	18 (11–30)	31 (14–66)	12 (7.4–19)	19 (9.0–41)
60 ~ 69	14 (6.3–31)	50 (22–114)	11 (6.3–20)	8.4 (2.2–32)

after 40 years for gBRCA1m and late 40 years for g*BRCA2*m, and few women received RRSO at the age recommended by the NCCN guidelines. With the insurance coverage of risk-reducing surgery in April 2020, the number of women with g*BRCA1/2*m undergoing RRSO is dramatically increasing. Accordingly, it has become important to provide appropriate information through genetic counseling and to consider the appropriate timing of RRSO for each case.

Therefore, we investigated the age of onset of breast and ovarian cancer in women with g*BRCA1/2*m in Japan [32]. First, as basic data, the current lifetime risk of ovarian cancer and breast cancer in the Japanese population is 1.6% and 10.9%, respectively, and the ratio of the incidence of breast cancer to ovarian cancer calculated from these values was found to be approximately 0.15. This analysis was performed using the database of the Japan Organization of Hereditary Breast and Ovarian Cancer (JOHBOC) national registry. The subjects were 3517 families with germline *BRCA* testing, 11.1% with g*BRCA1*m and 8.3% with g*BRCA2*m. Table 5.2 shows the onset age of ovarian cancer and the ratio of breast cancer to ovarian cancer, classified into g*BRCA1*m, g*BRCA2*m, and g*BRCA*wt (women without g*BRCA1/2*m) [32]. The onset age of ovarian cancer was 51.3 years for g*BRCA1*m, 58.3 years for g*BRCA2*m, and 53.8 years for g*BRCA*wt. Women with g*BRCA1*m developed ovarian cancer significantly younger than those with g*BRCA*wt. Notably, women with g*BRCA2*m developed the disease at a significantly older age than those with g*BRCA*wt. The risk of developing ovarian cancer in women with g*BRCA2*m was ten times higher than in the general population; however, the age of onset was later. A recent report from outside Japan, in a retrospective cohort study of patients diagnosed with high-grade serous carcinoma of ovary/fallopian tube/peritoneum, showed a significantly higher age at diagnosis in g*BRCA2*m compared to g*BRCA1*m (58.4 vs. 53.3 years; $P = 0.001$) [33].

It is important to note, however, in interpreting these results, that the subjects of the analysis were those who had undergone germline *BRCA* testing. The subjects included those with a family history of breast and ovarian cancer. Therefore, even if the subject did not have a mutation in the *BRCA1/2* gene, it is expected that those with mutation in other breast/ovarian cancer susceptibility gene would be included in the g*BRCA*wt group. The ratio of breast cancer to ovarian cancer was 0.52 for g*BRCA1*m, 0.15 for g*BRCA2*m, and 0.11 for g*BRCA*wt (Table 5.3) [34]. While the higher risk of ovarian cancer in g*BRCA1*m is to be expected, it is very interesting that the ratio in g*BRCA2*m was almost equal to that in the general population.

Table 5.2 Clinical characteristics of the ovarian cancer patients in the JOHBOC database

	g*BRCA*1m		g*BRCA*2m		g*BRCA*wt		
	n = 185		*n* = 42		*n* = 241		p-value
Histological subtype	n	%	n	%	n	%	*P*<0.001†
Serous carcinoma	138	74.6%	32	76.2%	125	51.9%	
Endomerioid carcinoma	14	7.6%	1	2.4%	25	10.4%	
Clearcell carcinoma	1	0.5%	1	2.4%	43	17.8%	
Mucinous carcinoma	1	0.5%	1	2.4%	10	4.1%	
Others	10	5.4%	2	4.8%	11	4.6%	
Unknown	21	11.4%	5	11.9%	27	11.2%	
FIGO stage							*p* = 0.018†
I	19	10.3%	5	11.9%	52	21.6%	
II	16	8.6%	2	4.8%	17	7.1%	
III	102	55.1%	23	54.8%	99	41.1%	
IV	26	14.1%	6	14.3%	42	17.4%	
Unknown	22	11.9%	6	14.3%	31	12.9%	
Personal breast cancer history							*p* = 0.18‡
Yes	54	29.2%	16	38.1%	60	24.9%	
No	131	70.8%	26	61.9%	181	75.1%	
Menopausal status							*P* = 0.001†
Premenopause	54	29.2%	6	14.3%	45	18.7%	
Postmenopause	90	48.6%	31	73.8%	181	75.1%	
Unknown	41	22.2%	5	11.9%	15	6.2%	
Age at diagnosis of OC							
Mean ± SD	51.3 ± 9.8		58.3 ± 9.3		53.8 ± 13.2		
Median	50		57.5		54		
Min	28		41		12		
Max	83		77		81		
p-value*	*p* = 0.039		*p* = 0.034		Ref.		

g germline, *m* mutation, *wt* wildtype, *OC* ovarian cancer, *ref.* reference
†Fisher's exact test (excluding unknown cases) ‡ Chi-square test
*T-test (vs. g*BRCA*wt)

Table 5.3 Difference in the number of ovarian cancer (OC) and breast cancer (BC) cases, and the ratio of OC to BC (number of OC patients/number of BC patients) by *BRCA* variant status

	g*BRCA1*m	g*BRCA*2m	g*BRCA*wt
No. of families	398	293	2826
No. of carriers	568	352	–
No. of ovarian cancer patients	334 (185†)	86 (42†)	497
No. of breast cancer patients	637 (373†)	590 (291†)	4444
Ovarian cancer prevalence*	0.84	0.29	0.18
Breast cancer prevalence*	1.60	2.01	1.57
Ratio of OC to BC	0.52‡ (0.50†)	0.15§ (0.14†)	0.11

g germline, *m* mutation, *wt* wild type, *OC* ovarian cancer, *BC* breast cancer
†Calculated only for carriers
‡$p < 0.0001$ (vs. g*BRCA*wt)
§$p = 0.037$ (vs. g*BRCA*wt)
*Per family

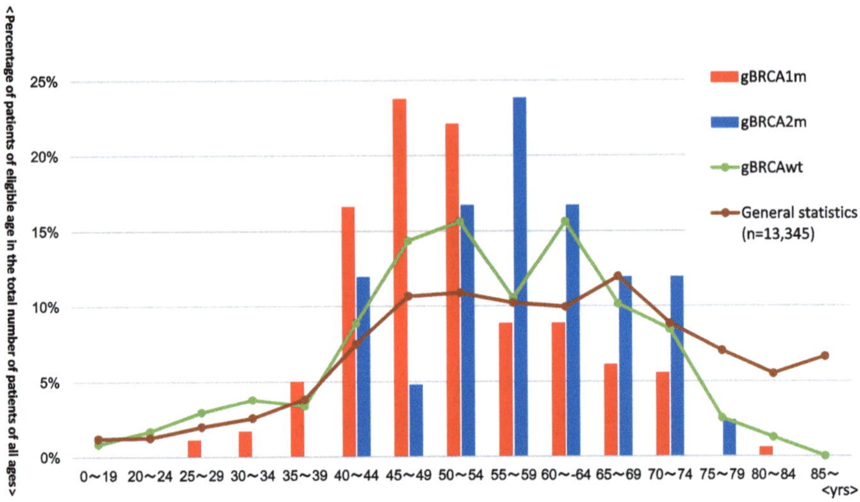

Fig. 5.1 Age distribution of ovarian cancer diagnosis by *BRCA1/2* mutation status in Japan

Figure 5.1 shows the onset age of ovarian cancer for each group [32]. Compared to women with g*BRCA1*m who developed ovarian cancer in their 20s, women with g*BRCA2*m did not develop ovarian cancer before the age of 40. This analysis provides details on the onset age of ovarian cancer in Japanese women with g*BRCA1/2*m and indicates that women with g*BRCA2*m may be able to wait until age 40 to perform RRSO. This Japanese data will allow for individualized genetic counseling for each mutated gene and current age. It will be possible to consider the best time to perform RRSO in accordance with the individual's life plan. However, the risk of breast cancer must also be considered in determining the age at which to perform RRSO. Regarding the onset age of breast cancer in g*BRCA1/2*m, Japanese data have shown that both patients with g*BRCA1*m and g*BRCA2*m have an increased risk of breast cancer starting in their 20s [21].

Since it has been reported that RRSO can reduce breast cancer risk by approximately 50%, genetic counseling should also provide accurate information on the risk of developing breast cancer in Japan before deciding when to perform RRSO. If individualized counseling on cancer risk can be provided based on Japanese data, the benefits for women who wish to have children are enormous, including the possibility of delaying the age at which RRSO should be performed.

5.10 Conclusion

The latest findings on RRSO were described, focusing on the management of aged patients with breast cancer. Although aged patients with breast cancer do not have the disadvantage of loss of fertility, their individual circumstances, including their physical condition due to breast cancer, the impact of treatment for breast cancer on their lives, and their attitudes toward their remaining lifetime, influence the decision to perform RRSO.

In addition, genetic counseling for women with g*BRCA1/2*m should ideally be based on Japanese data to provide individualized information. For each client, it is important to confirm their future life plans and onset age of HBOC-related cancer patients in the family. Finally, if the risk of developing cancer can be calculated specifically for *BRCA1/2* mutation type and genetic counseling can be based on scientific data from the Japanese population, the benefit to the *BRCA* mutation carriers in the family will be great.

References

1. Sekine M, Enomoto T. Precision medicine for hereditary tumors in gynecologic malignancies. J Obstet Gynaecol Res. 2021;47:2597–606.
2. Rebbeck TR, Kauff ND, Domchek SM. Meta-analysis of risk reduction estimates associated with risk-reducing salpingo-oophorectomy in BRCA1 or BRCA2 mutation carriers. J Natl Cancer Inst. 2009;101:80–7.
3. Marchetti C, De Felice F, Palaia I, Perniola G, Musella A, Musio D, Muzii L, Tombolini V, Panici PB. Risk-reducing salpingo-oophorectomy: a meta-analysis on impact on ovarian cancer risk and all cause mortality in BRCA 1 and BRCA 2 mutation carriers. BMC Womens Health. 2014;14:150.
4. Eleje GU, Eke AC, Ezebialu IU, Ikechebelu JI, Ugwu EO, Okonkwo OO. Risk-reducing bilateral salpingo-oophorectomy in women with BRCA1 or BRCA2 mutations. Cochrane Database Syst Rev. 2018;8:Cd012464.
5. Wang Y, Song Z, Zhang S, Wang X, Li P. Risk-reducing salpingo-oophorectomy and breast cancer risk in BRCA1 or BRCA2 mutation carriers: a systematic review and meta-analysis. Eur J Surg Oncol. 2022;48:1209–16.
6. Gaba F, Blyuss O, Tan A, Munblit D, Oxley S, Khan K, Legood R, Manchanda R. Breast cancer risk and breast-cancer-specific mortality following risk-reducing salpingo-oophorectomy in BRCA carriers: a systematic review and meta-analysis. Cancers. 2023;15:1625.
7. Domchek SM, Friebel TM, Singer CF, Evans DG, Lynch HT, Isaacs C, Garber JE, Neuhausen SL, Matloff E, Eeles R, et al. Association of risk-reducing surgery in BRCA1 or BRCA2 mutation carriers with cancer risk and mortality. JAMA. 2010;304:967–75.
8. Marchetti C, De Felice F, Boccia S, Sassu C, Di Donato V, Perniola G, Palaia I, Monti M, Muzii L, Tombolini V, et al. Hormone replacement therapy after prophylactic risk-reducing salpingo-oophorectomy and breast cancer risk in BRCA1 and BRCA2 mutation carriers: a meta-analysis. Crit Rev Oncol Hematol. 2018;132:111–5.
9. Gordhandas S, Norquist BM, Pennington KP, Yung RL, Laya MB, Swisher EM. Hormone replacement therapy after risk reducing salpingo-oophorectomy in patients with BRCA1 or BRCA2 mutations; a systematic review of risks and benefits. Gynecol Oncol. 2019;153:192–200.
10. Xiao YL, Wang K, Liu Q, Li J, Zhang X, Li HY. Risk reduction and survival benefit of risk-reducing salpingo-oophorectomy in hereditary breast cancer: meta-analysis and systematic review. Clin Breast Cancer. 2019;19:e48–65.
11. Stroot IAS, Brouwer J, Bart J, Hollema H, Stommel-Jenner DJ, Wagner MM, van Doorn HC, de Hullu JA, Gaarenstroom KN, Beurden M, et al. High-grade serous carcinoma at risk-reducing salpingo-oophorectomy in asymptomatic carriers of BRCA1/2 pathogenic variants: prevalence and clinical factors. J Clin Oncol Off J Am Soc Clin Oncol. 2023;41:2523–35.

12. Finch AP, Lubinski J, Møller P, Singer CF, Karlan B, Senter L, Rosen B, Maehle L, Ghadirian P, Cybulski C, et al. Impact of oophorectomy on cancer incidence and mortality in women with a BRCA1 or BRCA2 mutation. J Clin Oncol Off J Am Soc Clin Oncol. 2014;32:1547–53.
13. Casey MJ, Synder C, Bewtra C, Narod SA, Watson P, Lynch HT. Intra-abdominal carcinomatosis after prophylactic oophorectomy in women of hereditary breast ovarian cancer syndrome kindreds associated with BRCA1 and BRCA2 mutations. Gynecol Oncol. 2005;97:457–67.
14. Harmsen MG, Piek JMJ, Bulten J, Casey MJ, Rebbeck TR, Mourits MJ, Greene MH, Slangen BFM, van Beurden M, Massuger L, et al. Peritoneal carcinomatosis after risk-reducing surgery in BRCA1/2 mutation carriers. Cancer. 2018;124:952–9.
15. Finch A, Beiner M, Lubinski J, Lynch HT, Moller P, Rosen B, Murphy J, Ghadirian P, Friedman E, Foulkes WD, et al. Salpingo-oophorectomy and the risk of ovarian, fallopian tube, and peritoneal cancers in women with a BRCA1 or BRCA2 mutation. JAMA. 2006;296:185–92.
16. Steenbeek MP, van Bommel MHD, Bulten J, Hulsmann JA, Bogaerts J, Garcia C, Cun HT, Lu KH, van Beekhuizen HJ, Minig L, et al. Risk of peritoneal carcinomatosis after risk-reducing salpingo-oophorectomy: a systematic review and individual patient data meta-analysis. J Clin Oncol Off J Am Soc Clin Oncol. 2022;40:1879–91.
17. Zakhour M, Danovitch Y, Lester J, Rimel BJ, Walsh CS, Li AJ, Karlan BY, Cass I. Occult and subsequent cancer incidence following risk-reducing surgery in BRCA mutation carriers. Gynecol Oncol. 2016;143:231–5.
18. Heemskerk-Gerritsen BA, Seynaeve C, van Asperen CJ, Ausems MG, Collée JM, van Doorn HC, Gomez Garcia EB, Kets CM, van Leeuwen FE, Meijers-Heijboer HE, et al. Breast cancer risk after salpingo-oophorectomy in healthy BRCA1/2 mutation carriers: revisiting the evidence for risk reduction. J Natl Cancer Inst. 2015;107
19. Choi YH, Terry MB, Daly MB, MacInnis RJ, Hopper JL, Colonna S, Buys SS, Andrulis IL, John EM, Kurian AW, et al. Association of risk-reducing salpingo-oophorectomy with breast cancer risk in women with BRCA1 and BRCA2 pathogenic variants. JAMA Oncol. 2021;7:585–92.
20. Kauff ND, Domchek SM, Friebel TM, Robson ME, Lee J, Garber JE, Isaacs C, Evans DG, Lynch H, Eeles RA, et al. Risk-reducing salpingo-oophorectomy for the prevention of BRCA1- and BRCA2-associated breast and gynecologic cancer: a multicenter, prospective study. J Clin Oncol Off J Am Soc Clin Oncol. 2008;26:1331–7.
21. Okano M, Nomizu T, Tachibana K, Nagatsuka M, Matsuzaki M, Katagata N, Ohtake T, Yokoyama S, Arai M, Nakamura S. The relationship between BRCA-associated breast cancer and age factors: an analysis of the Japanese HBOC consortium database. J Hum Genet. 2021;66:307–14.
22. Tutt ANJ, Garber JE, Kaufman B, Viale G, Fumagalli D, Rastogi P, Gelber RD, de Azambuja E, Fielding A, Balmaña J, et al. Adjuvant olaparib for patients with BRCA1- or BRCA2-mutated breast cancer. N Engl J Med. 2021;384:2394–405.
23. Sessa C, Balmaña J, Bober SL, Cardoso MJ, Colombo N, Curigliano G, Domchek SM, Evans DG, Fischerova D, Harbeck N, et al. Risk reduction and screening of cancer in hereditary breast-ovarian cancer syndromes: ESMO clinical practice guideline. Ann Oncol. 2023;34:33–47.
24. Huber D, Seitz S, Kast K, Emons G, Ortmann O. Use of oral contraceptives in BRCA mutation carriers and risk for ovarian and breast cancer: a systematic review. Arch Gynecol Obstet. 2020;301:875–84.
25. van Bommel MHD, IntHout J, Veldmate G, Kets CM, de Hullu JA, van Altena AM, Harmsen MG. Contraceptives and cancer risks in BRCA1/2 pathogenic variant carriers: a systematic review and meta-analysis. Hum Reprod Update. 2023;29:197–217.
26. Narod SA, Risch H, Moslehi R, Dørum A, Neuhausen S, Olsson H, Provencher D, Radice P, Evans G, Bishop S, et al. Oral contraceptives and the risk of hereditary ovarian cancer. Hereditary ovarian cancer clinical study group. N Engl J Med. 1998;339:424–8.
27. NCCN Clinical practice guidelines in oncology: genetic/familial high-risk assessment: breast and ovarian, 2024.

28. Antoniou A, Pharoah PD, Narod S, Risch HA, Eyfjord JE, Hopper JL, Loman N, Olsson H, Johannsson O, Borg A, et al. Average risks of breast and ovarian cancer associated with BRCA1 or BRCA2 mutations detected in case series unselected for family history: a combined analysis of 22 studies. Am J Hum Genet. 2003;72:1117–30.
29. Sekine M, Nishino K, Enomoto T. Differences in ovarian and other cancers risks by population and BRCA mutation location. Genes. 2021;12
30. Sekine M, Nishino K, Enomoto T. BRCA genetic test and risk-reducing salpingo-oophorectomy for hereditary breast and ovarian cancer: state-of-the-art. Cancers. 2021;13:2562.
31. Nomura H, Sekine M, Yokoyama S, Arai M, Enomoto T, Takeshima N, Nakamura S. Clinical background and outcomes of risk-reducing salpingo-oophorectomy for hereditary breast and ovarian cancers in Japan. Int J Clin Oncol. 2019;24:1105–10.
32. Sekine M, Enomoto T, Arai M, Den H, Nomura H, Ikeuchi T, Nakamura S. Differences in age at diagnosis of ovarian cancer for each BRCA mutation type in Japan: optimal timing to carry out risk-reducing salpingo-oophorectomy. J Gynecol Oncol. 2022;33:e46.
33. Marchetti C, Ataseven B, Cassani C, Sassu CM, Congedo L, D'Indinosante M, Cappuccio S, Rhiem K, Hahnen E, Lucci Cordisco E, et al. Ovarian cancer onset across different BRCA mutation types: a view to a more tailored approach for BRCA mutated patients. Int J Gynecol Cancer. 2023;33:257–62.
34. Sekine M, Enomoto T, Arai M, Yokoyama S, Nomura H, Nishino K, Ikeuchi T, Kuriyama Y, Nakamura S. Correlation between the risk of ovarian cancer and BRCA recurrent pathogenic variants in Japan. J Hum Genet. 2022;67:267–72.

Chapter 6
"Gene Awareness"

Arisa Ueki

Abstract The introduction of multigene panel (MGP) testing has enabled the simultaneous analysis of multiple genes. In addition, the broader application of tumor profiling targeting germline and somatic variants has facilitated fewer oversights. A definitive diagnosis of the causative gene in hereditary tumors is endurance, effect on the family, and predictiveness of cancer onset. In addition, managing patients with hereditary tumors necessitates meticulous care. Moreover, genetic information holds potential for guiding subsequent treatment selection and providing actionable insights into diseases. Clinicians might be reluctant to definitively diagnose hereditary tumors, given the implications on family members; however, such hesitancy is unwarranted. We introduce the term "gene awareness" inspired by breast awareness to underscore our commitment to providing knowledge and awareness of genetic diagnosis. We aim to disseminate "gene awareness" among healthcare providers, patients, and the general population. This initiative aims to develop knowledge of hereditary tumors and the benefits of genetic information among medical professionals, enabling them to provide informed recommendations to patients, and potentially influencing public health awareness. By expanding "gene awareness" nationwide, we hope to increase opportunities and demand for consulting about hereditary tumors without hesitation.

Keywords "Gene awareness" · Hereditary tumors · Genetic diagnosis · Genetic testing · Multigene panel (MGP) testing · Syndrome-specific genetic testing

A. Ueki (✉)
Department of Clinical Genetic Oncology, Cancer Institute Hospital of Japanese Foundation for Cancer Research, Tokyo, Japan
e-mail: Arisa.ueki@jfcr.or.jp

A. Sakurai et al. (eds.), *Practical Guide to Hereditary Breast and Ovarian Cancer II*, https://doi.org/10.1007/978-981-96-4329-5_6

6.1 Introduction

The use of next-generation sequencing has ushered in a novel era of affordable and rapid genetic analysis, notably impacting our understanding of hereditary tumors. The introduction of multigene panel (MGP) testing has revolutionized genetic testing by enabling the simultaneous assessment of multiple genes. In addition, molecular tumor profiling is a type of epoch-making method for determining therapeutic targets. The use of tumor profiling as biomarkers has emerged as a novel approach to the construction of clinical treatment strategies. The capabilities of tumor profiling, targeting both germline and somatic variants, have expanded significantly with the advent of cancer genomic profiling tests, leading to fewer oversights. The utilization of whole exome sequence and whole genome sequence for practical use makes it evident that inspection technology continues to witness rapid technological advancements.

A definitive diagnosis of the causative gene of a hereditary tumor is enduring, impacting the family, while also serving as a predictive indicator for cancer onset. Consequently, careful consideration is warranted when managing patients with a genetic diagnosis of hereditary tumors. However, genetic information holds promise for guiding treatment decisions and offering actionable insights into diseases. When a germline pathogenic variant associated with a hereditary tumor-related gene is detected as germline findings from tumor profiling, it can serve as a valuable resource in treatment selection strategies for the individual patient. Clinicians may be reluctant to make a definitive diagnosis of hereditary tumors, given the concomitant effects on family members. Understanding by clinicians and patients that hereditary tumor-related genes provide vital insights for primary cancer prevention in family members can facilitate appropriate medical intervention. A comprehensive understanding of hereditary tumors equips clinicians with valuable tools derived from tumor profiling information, enabling them to deliver enhanced medical care to their patients.

We have introduced an initiative named "gene awareness." Genetic information obtained from patients with cancer is increasingly prevalent in guiding their treatment and preventive measures. Particularly in the field of oncology, a rising trend is observed in medical professionals leveraging genetic information to identify suitable treatment and prevention strategies.

"Gene awareness" is an initiative to enhance awareness of hereditary tumors among medical professionals and Japanese society, with the aim of optimizing the utilization of genetic information for treatment and family health.

6.2 Definition of "Gene Awareness"

We have coined the term "gene awareness," drawing inspiration from breast awareness, which encompasses breast cancer self-examination. We envision "gene awareness" to achieve the same level of recognition among the general public as breast awareness. Our proposal extends to everyone, including not only medical professionals but also the general population, encouraging the application of "gene awareness" to leverage genetic diagnosis for treatment and prevention.

The rationales behind improving "gene awareness" are given below:

1. To advance knowledge, skills, and awareness in clinical genetics without discrimination through specialized training fostering multidisciplinary medical care across various medical departments.
2. To raise awareness regarding genetic diagnosis within the medical field and society at large, by disseminating accurate information on hereditary diseases.

Each genetic diagnosis carries the importance of accurately assessing and managing the risk for relatives. Recognizing that disclosing germline findings from cancer genomic profile testing can potentially reduce cancer-related fatalities through medical intervention within families is imperative. Therefore, genetic counseling plays a pivotal role in consolidating accurate information for patients and their families, aiding in understanding and contributing to the reduction of cancer mortality. We believe that educating clinicians about hereditary tumors and the importance of genetic interventions through "gene awareness" activities will improve the health outcomes of unaffected relatives.

Our efforts in promoting "gene awareness" initiatives have led to the establishment of a medical system based on genetic diagnosis within the hospital as a collaborative endeavor among various medical teams. This project is supported by the Department of Clinical Genetics Oncology, Genomic Medicine, Gynecologic Oncology, Genitourinary Oncology, Medical Oncology, Breast Oncology Center, Gastroenterology Center, Division of Pathology, Diagnostic Imaging Center, The Department of Advanced Medical Development, Department of Nursing, Pharmacy, Clinical Laboratory Center, and Administrative Department in the Cancer Institute Hospital. We have created posters for the "gene awareness" team, and we utilize them for disseminating information within our hospital (Fig. 6.1). In addition, we conduct regular cross-disciplinary meetings to exchange insights on hereditary tumors.

In genetic counseling, we strive to offer the necessary psychosocial support to transform genetic diagnosis into positive information. Unfortunately, some patients and their families perceive genetic diagnosis as bad news. We expect to play an important role in raising awareness within the society concerning genetic information, refraining from labeling it as inherently "good" or "bad," but rather as an integral aspect of an individual. Therefore, we have set the overarching goal of the "gene awareness" project: "Everyone possesses genetic variations."

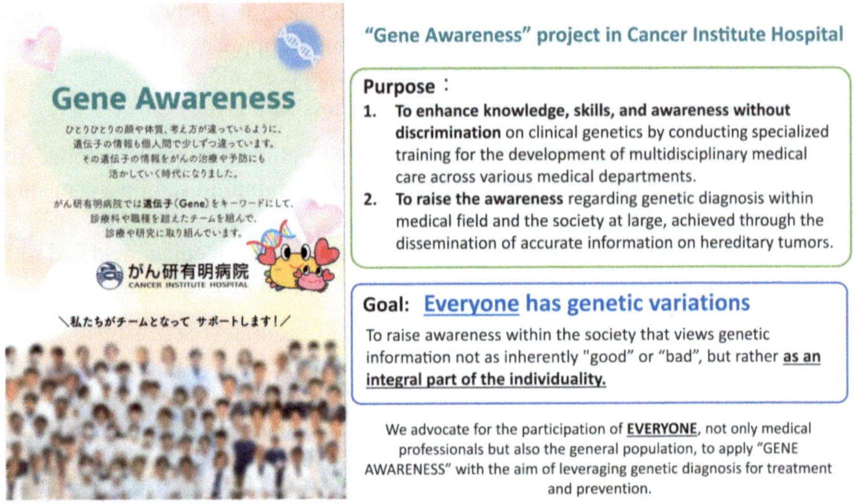

Fig. 6.1 Purpose and goals of our "gene awareness" project. We believe that informing clinicians about hereditary tumors and the importance of genetic interventions through "gene awareness" activities will improve the health of unaffected relatives

6.3 Changes Surrounding Genetic Testing for Hereditary Tumors

Traditionally, genetic counseling for hereditary tumors relied on assessments of past medical and family histories. However, in recent years, a notable increase has been observed in genetic diagnoses involving hereditary tumor-related genes through cancer profiling tests, often referred to as secondary findings or germline findings. Additionally, the introduction of *BRCA1/2* genetic testing as a companion diagnostic for PARP inhibitor treatment is anticipated to contribute to a rise in diagnoses of hereditary breast and ovarian cancer (HBOC) in Japan. Since 2020, our hospital has observed approximately 700–800 patients undergoing *BRCA1/2* genetic testing annually.

In the near future, a notable challenge lies in efficiently conducting presymptomatic diagnosis for relatives who have not yet developed the disease and facilitating their access to appropriate medical intervention for cancer prevention. We have experienced numerous cases where patients seek genetic counseling for various reasons.

Genetic testing methods include syndrome-specific genetic testing as the classical genetic testing, such as *BRCA1/2* genetic testing, which targets the most suspicious hereditary cancer for the patient, and MGP testing, which simultaneously assesses multiple hereditary cancer-related genes. In recent years, there has been a notable increase in the diagnoses of hereditary cancer-related genes through cancer genome profiling tests, as germline findings. Our hospital's experience indicates that germline findings are detected in approximately 6–7% of cancer genomic profiling tests (in press).

There are a wide variety of hereditary tumors, with related tumors occurring in multiple organs. As a result of MGP testing, various hereditary tumor-related genes are increasingly being revealed. For instance, gynecological-related tumors such as ovarian and endometrial cancers are associated with multiple hereditary tumor syndromes. Similarly, breast-related tumors, including early-onset breast cancer, encompass a diverse range of hereditary tumor syndromes. Thus, a single kind of tumor can lead to the diagnosis of various hereditary tumor syndromes. Consequently, even if the *BRCA1/2* gene test yields negative results, patients may warrant consideration for other hereditary tumor-related genes. We are currently navigating an era where proficiency in both syndrome-specific genetic testing and MGP testing is essential.

6.4 Multigene Panel (MGP) Testing

MGP testing is a methodology that simultaneously analyzes a predefined set of genes associated with hereditary cancers. Its introduction is anticipated to broaden the scope of diagnoses for individuals with pathogenic variants in hereditary cancer-related genes, which might have remained undetected through conventional syndrome-specific genetic testing. Kurian et al. reported that MGP testing replaced *BRCA1/2*-syndrome-specific genetic testing in 2014 [1]. The proliferation of MGP testing is expected to reduce the number of missed diagnoses of hereditary tumors (Fig. 6.2). At our hospital, the utilization of MGP testing has demonstrated a consistent annual increase (Fig. 6.3).

However, it is imperative to recognize that the adoption of MGP testing may lead to an upsurge in cases involving unexpected and rare hereditary tumors that were not previously considered. Consequently, MGP testing should be approached with caution, considering the latest guidelines for managing rare hereditary cancer-related genes. The 2020 edition of the NCCN guidelines [2, 3] underscored a significant paradigm shift, recommending MGP testing as the primary genetic testing modality.

According to the guidelines of the American College of Medical Genetics and Genomics (ACMG) [4], the results of genetic testing are classified into five categories: "pathogenic," "likely pathogenic," "benign," "likely benign," and "variant of uncertain significance (VUS)." The VUS classification indicates that the pathogenicity cannot be determined, although there are some variants in the gene. It should be noted that genetic management based solely on VUS results is not recommended.

With MGP targeting multiple hereditary cancer-related genes, the increasing prevalence of MGP testing is anticipated to coincide with a rise in the identification of rare hereditary cancer-related genes classified as VUS. Consequently, additional confirmatory measures may be required to ensure accurate interpretation [5–8]. It is

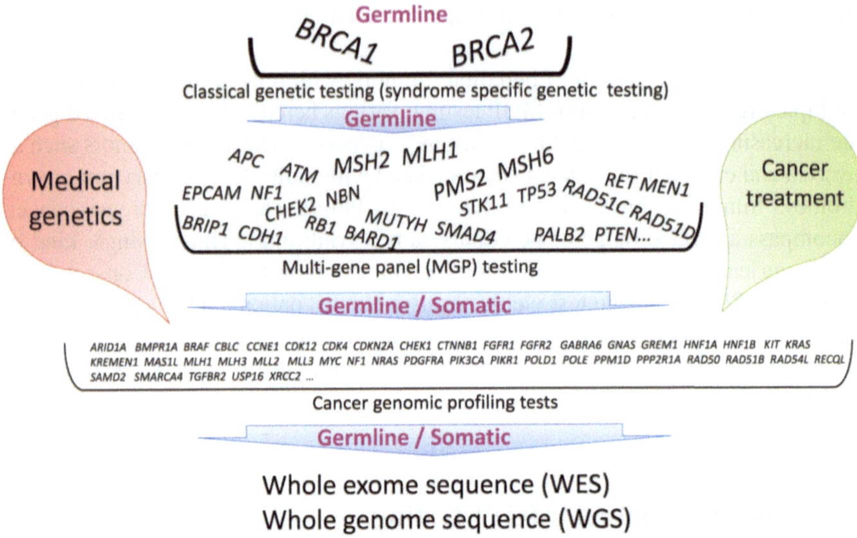

Fig. 6.2 Transitions in genetic testing methods. MGP testing has reduced the number of missed genetic diagnoses from syndrome-specific testing, which assumes a specific hereditary tumor. An era in which whole exome sequence (WES)/whole genome sequence (WGS) will be utilized is expected in the near future

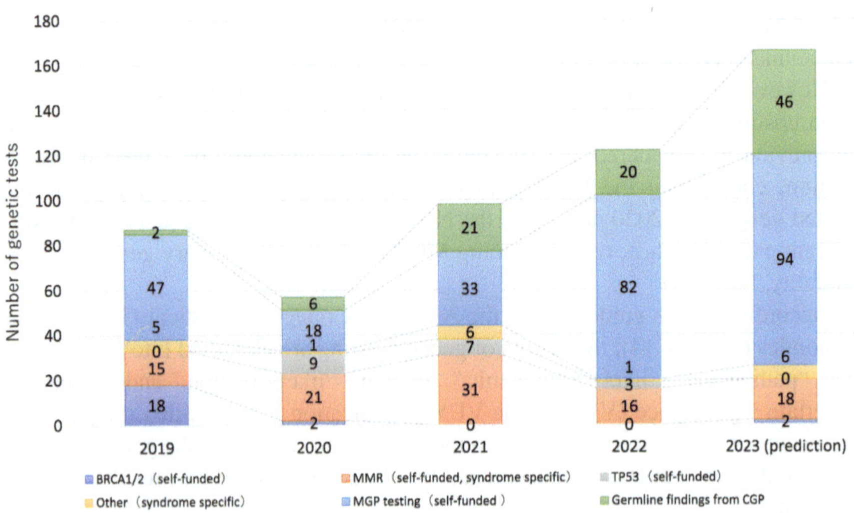

Fig. 6.3 Number of genetic tests performed on probands (excludes BRACAnalysis). The number of multigene panel (MGP) tests is on the rise. The number of genetic confirmation tests after cancer gene panel (CGP) testing is also increasing

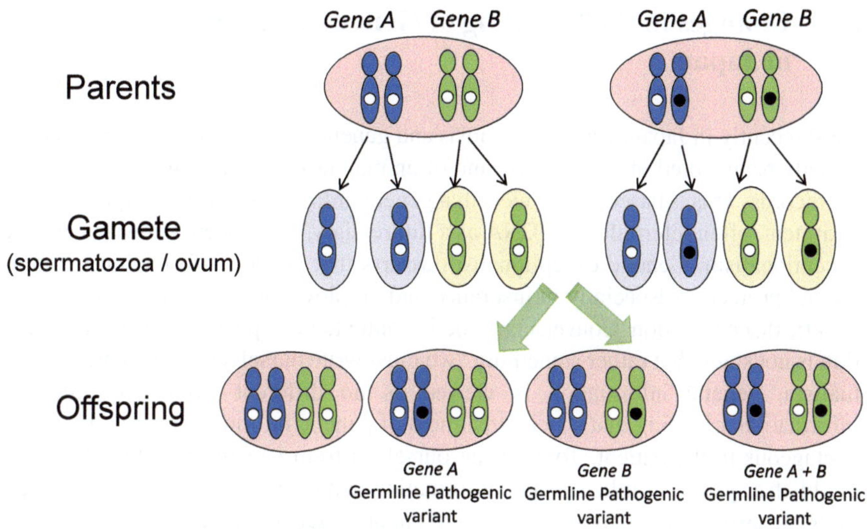

Fig. 6.4 Genetic forms of double heterozygote. Double heterozygotes have a 75% chance of being passed on to the next generation

essential to acknowledge that the interpretation of VUS may evolve over time as new data emerges. Thus, medical professionals involved in genetics must continually gather information based on the latest evidence to inform patient health management effectively.

MGP testing has the potential to reveal pathogenic variants across multiple genes, thereby complicating the assessment of genetic risks and making it difficult to make risk management decisions. For instance, carriers of two pathogenic variants, known as double heterozygotes, exhibit a 75% likelihood of passing on these variants to the next generation, rather than the typical 50% (Fig. 6.4). Genetic counseling for families of patients identified as carriers of multiple pathogenic variants necessitates careful assessment of genetic risk.

Furthermore, it is necessary to conduct thorough preliminary investigations regarding commercially available MGP testing as there are variations among different companies concerning the genes targeted for analysis, and not all targeted genes are clinically compatible. For these reasons, MGP testing must be accompanied by both pre- and post-test genetic counseling provided by professionals based on genetic expertise [3, 9]. As a result of MGP testing, various causative genes have been identified. Therefore, the implementation system of genetic medicine is also in a period of transition. Consequently, it is important to accurately interpret the results and communicate them effectively with the patient's family. For the advancement of cancer genomic medicine, the dissemination and communication of germline findings are pivotal. Equally important is the provision of accurate information, and the establishment of a trusting relationship, accompanied by psychosocial support for patients and their families.

6.5 Changes in the Handling of Genetic Information in Japan

Until recently in Japan, genetic diagnosis and genetic counseling records have traditionally been stored in paper charts and often managed independently within medical records. This is based on the view that genetic information should require special treatment, often referred to as "DNA as a future diary," as concept known as genetic exceptionalism. Genetic exceptionalism asserts that genetic information warrants special protection especially in insurance and employment, due to the potential for genetic discrimination. Conversely, genetic contextualism posits that DNA information is not static, but rather something "we must write ourselves." In genetic contextualism, genetic information is viewed as no different from other medical information, claiming that special treatment of genetic information would be disadvantageous to the patient. To extricate ourselves from genetic exceptionalism and establish a system to utilize genetic information in medical care is necessary. As part of "gene awareness" activities, we aim to enhance genetic literacy to eradicate discrimination based on genetic changes among all hospital staff, not just medical staff. We anticipate that reforming the awareness of all staff who interact with patients and their families will lead to "gene awareness" among the general public. To achieve "gene awareness," we provide concise e-learning training to all hospital staff on personal information protection and the appropriate handling of genetic information. Through nationwide dissemination of "gene awareness," we aspire to increase opportunities and demand for consulting about hereditary tumors without hesitation.

6.6 Spreading the "Gene Awareness" Effect on Society

What sets "gene awareness" apart as innovative and unique is its inclusive approach, targeting not only medical professionals but society as a whole. By fostering "gene awareness," we aim to cultivate an understanding of hereditary tumors, and the advantages of genetic information among medical professionals, empowering them to provide informed recommendations to patients. This, in turn, has the potential to influence public health awareness positively. Through widespread dissemination of the "gene awareness" keyword, we envision that familiarity with genetic information will permeate to the general public. Once "gene awareness" is successfully disseminated in patients with cancer, our focus will shift toward implementing initiatives aimed at the general public.

The enactment of the "Comprehensive and Systematic Promotion of Measures to Ensure High-Quality and Appropriate Genomic Medicine for Citizens to Receive with Confidence Act (Law No. 57 of 2023)" in 2023 in Japan aims to comprehensively and systematically promote genomic medicine policies. In the near future, opportunities to learn more about genetic literacy will be provided to medical professionals, patients, and the general public using "gene awareness" as a keyword.

6.7 Conclusion

In recent years, various genetic tests have been introduced into clinical practice, and the means for genetic diagnosis have diversified. There are increasing opportunities to identify various causative genes of hereditary tumors. It is important to capitalize on these advancements by leveraging genetic diagnosis for the treatment and prevention of patients with cancer themselves, and in the maintenance of the health of their relatives.

The initiative we propose, "gene awareness," seeks to enhance awareness of genetic diagnosis. We advocate for a shift in perspective where genetic variants are not treated as inherently good or bad. If we examine about 20,000 genes in one person through whole-genome analysis, we will find changes in not just one or two, but dozens of genes. It is crucial to recognize that the relevance of these changes to the disease varies depending on the disease and remains partially understood. We work with the hope of creating an ideal society where genetic changes and variants are treated as facets of individuality, devoid of stigma or impediment.

We advocate for the promotion of "gene awareness" as a positive endeavor. By realizing and deepening our understanding of the information obtained from genes, we endeavor to catalyze societal change. It is also important to improve the understanding of the doctors across various clinical departments, ensuring comprehensive support for individuals affected by hereditary tumors. Though ongoing efforts to cultivate understanding and change perceptions, we aim to foster an environment where doctors involved in genetic information refrain from adopting negative attitudes toward patients.

References

1. Kurian AW, Ward KC, Hamilton AS, Deapen DM, Abrahamse P, Bondarenko I, et al. Uptake, results, and outcomes of germline multiple-gene sequencing after diagnosis of breast cancer. JAMA Oncol. 2018;4(8):1066–72.
2. Daly MB, Pilarski R, Yurgelun MB, Berry MP, Buys SS, Dickson P, et al. NCCN guidelines insights: genetic/familial high-risk assessment: breast, ovarian, and pancreatic, version 1.2020. J Natl Compr Cancer Netw. 2020;18(4):380–91.
3. Network NCC. NCCN clinical practice guideline in oncology, genetic / familial high-risk assessment: Colorectal, version1. 2020. [Available from: https://www.nccn.org/professionals/physician_gls/pdf/genetics_colon.pdf.
4. Richards S, Aziz N, Bale S, Bick D, Das S, Gastier-Foster J, et al. Standards and guidelines for the interpretation of sequence variants: a joint consensus recommendation of the American College of Medical Genetics and Genomics and the Association for Molecular Pathology. Genet Med. 2015;17(5):405–24.
5. Chang J, Seng S, Yoo J, Equivel P, Lum SS. Clinical management of patients at risk for hereditary breast cancer with variants of uncertain significance in the era of multigene panel testing. Ann Surg Oncol. 2019;26(10):3389–96.
6. Ndugga-Kabuye MK, Issaka RB. Inequities in multi-gene hereditary cancer testing: lower diagnostic yield and higher VUS rate in individuals who identify as Hispanic, African or Asian and Pacific Islander as compared to European. Fam Cancer. 2019;18(4):465–9.

7. Tsaousis GN, Papadopoulou E, Apessos A, Agiannitopoulos K, Pepe G, Kampouri S, et al. Analysis of hereditary cancer syndromes by using a panel of genes: novel and multiple pathogenic mutations. BMC Cancer. 2019;19(1):535.
8. Yurgelun MB, Allen B, Kaldate RR, Bowles KR, Judkins T, Kaushik P, et al. Identification of a variety of mutations in cancer predisposition genes in patients with suspected lynch syndrome. Gastroenterology. 2015;149(3):604–13.e20.
9. Network NCC. NCCN Clinical Practice Guidelines in Oncology. Genetic / Familial High-Risk Assessment: Breast, Ovarian, and Pancreatic version1, 2021. [Available from: https://www.nccn.org/professionals/physician_gls/pdf/genetics_bop.pdf.

Chapter 7
HBOC Guidebook for Patients and the Public

Yusuke Kobayashi

Abstract The social landscape surrounding hereditary breast and ovarian cancer (HBOC) in Japan has changed significantly since insurance coverage for part of its management began in April 2020. The introduction of poly(ADP-ribose) polymerase (PARP) inhibitors and their companion diagnostics has further expanded HBOC diagnosis, necessitating adaptation among healthcare providers unfamiliar with genetic diagnostics. In response, the Japan Organization of Hereditary Breast and Ovarian Cancer (JOHBOC) released the Guidelines for Diagnosis and Treatment of Hereditary Breast and Ovarian Cancer 2021 to standardize HBOC management. However, these guidelines, designed for medical professionals, were difficult for the general public to understand. To address this gap, JOHBOC and the Research on the Development of a Preemptive Medical Care Delivery System for Hereditary Tumors Using Genome Information group, supported by the Health and Labour Sciences Research Grant, developed a new guidebook tailored for patients and the public. A key feature of this guidebook is its emphasis on Patient and Public Involvement (PPI), a concept originally developed in the United Kingdom, which promotes collaboration with patients and the public in healthcare research and policy. The guidebook was created through extensive engagement with affected individuals, including patients, genetic counselors, and healthcare providers. A questionnaire survey collected input from 46 respondents, and four opinion-exchange meetings involving 36 participants were held. Ultimately, 82 members of the public contributed to the guidebook's development, ensuring that the content was accessible and aligned with the needs of those affected by HBOC. To maximize its reach and usability, the guidebook was structured in a Q&A format, addressing common concerns and misconceptions about HBOC. A notable example is the discussion on communicating an HBOC diagnosis to minor children, which underwent multiple revisions based on public feedback to ensure clarity and practical applicability. Furthermore, efforts were made to make the guidebook affordable and portable, with a title and format

Y. Kobayashi (✉)
Department of Obstetrics and Gynecology, Institute of Medicine, University of Tsukuba, Ibaraki, Japan
e-mail: kobayashi@md.tsukuba.ac.jp

A. Sakurai et al. (eds.), *Practical Guide to Hereditary Breast and Ovarian Cancer II*, https://doi.org/10.1007/978-981-96-4329-5_7

designed to encourage widespread use. The development of this guidebook has also provided valuable insights for healthcare professionals, reinforcing the importance of clear, empathetic communication in genetic counseling. Feedback from both medical professionals and the public highlighted the guidebook's role in fostering a shared understanding of HBOC, ultimately bridging the gap between medical knowledge and the lived experiences of patients and their families.

Keywords Hereditary breast and ovarian cancer · Patient and public involvement · Guidebook

7.1 Background to the Publication of the Guidebook for the Public

The social environment surrounding hereditary breast and ovarian cancer (HBOC) has changed significantly since part of HBOC management was covered by insurance in April 2020. Furthermore, with the clinical development of poly(ADP-ribose) polymerase inhibitors and the spread of their companion diagnoses, the opportunities to diagnose HBOC have increased rapidly and clinicians who were not previously familiar with the genetic diagnosis must now adapt to this situation. Under these circumstances, the Japan Organization of Hereditary Breast and Ovarian Cancer (JOHBOC) published the "Guidelines for Diagnosis and Treatment of Hereditary Breast and Ovarian Cancer 2021" in July 2021 to promote and normalize HBOC management. The guidelines were designed to comply with the "Guidebook for Diagnosis and Treatment of Hereditary Breast and Ovarian Cancer Syndrome 2017" and reflect the diverse values of individuals with BRCA pathogenic variants and healthcare providers, and to be used for decision-making. Particular emphasis was placed on considering the values and wishes of the person concerned. Two patients with cancer and one without cancer participated in the decision-making meetings to develop a set of recommendations. Literature and questionnaires regarding patient values and wishes were collected for all clinical questions (CQs). Recommendations were discussed at the decision-making meeting using the Evidence to Decision frameworks of the GRADE system to reflect patient values and intentions. The guidelines, which were written by experts in each field based on a precise algorithm, were educational and practical for medical practitioners; however, the content was difficult for the general public to understand because it was intended for medical practitioners. Therefore, a new guidebook for the general public was proposed by JOHBOC and the "Research on the development of a preemptive medical care delivery system for hereditary tumors using genome information" group of the Health and Labor Sciences Research Grant (Comprehensive Research Project for the Promotion of Cancer Control and Prevention).

7.2 Patient and Public Involvement Emphasized in the Creation of the Guidebook

The perspective shared by all members of the committee in preparing the guidebook was the desire to deliver a book that would be appreciated by all people affected by HBOC and their families. Specifically, the members hoped that this guidebook would be read and used widely by the general public, and passed on from person to person, to reach those who have "questions or concerns" in their daily lives. If the affected individuals would carry this guidebook with them, the medical community would need to be prepared to respond, and both groups would increase their understanding of HBOC. Based on these wishes, our policy in preparing this guidebook was (1) not to omit or change the words used by medical professionals in HBOC practice, but to present the reasons "why we use those words" as clearly as possible, and to explain that they can be correctly conveyed and understood, and (2) to provide answers in such a way that the reader feels as if he or she is talking to their doctor so the patient can think positively and not be overwhelmed by their dilemma. In creating this guidebook for the public in a Q&A format, we emphasized Patient and Public Involvement (PPI), a concept first adopted in the United Kingdom, which states that "research should not be conducted for or about the patient or the public, but with the patient or the public, or by the patient or the public." Specifically, the first step is "patients/citizens becoming research participants," such as participating in a clinical trial. The second stage is "the sharing of information and knowledge of research results by researchers with society after the research is completed," which includes providing information, such as clinical trial results to subjects and patient groups, which is known as "engagement." The third step is "involvement," meaning that patients and citizens are involved in planning, designing, managing, evaluating, and disseminating results as "research partners." This also includes active involvement as stakeholders in planning, monitoring, and evaluating healthcare-related policies, as well as considering solutions to various medical issues outside of the research field. Placing the greatest importance on introducing the concept of PPI into the guidebook, the original questions were collected, not only from physicians but also from genetic counselors and certified nurses who are consulted during genetic counseling, and a questionnaire was also sent to those affected to obtain their real voices. As a result, there were 46 respondents to the questionnaire, all of whom submitted draft questions. In preparing the answers, we not only strived to make the answers clear for the readers but also included the opinions of the patients and fellow citizens by holding four opinion-exchange meetings (total 10 h, total 36 persons). As a result, 82 members of the general public and concerned citizens participated in the preparation of this document.

7.3 Featured Question and Answer

Through the above PPI initiatives, the medical members of the committee prepared answers to the questions, which reflected the opinions of the people affected as well as the general public. The first three chapters were entitled "What to Know about HBOC," "What to Know if diagnosed with HBOC," and "What to Know about precautions in daily life" (Figure). The Q&A was developed within these themes. Here, a characteristic Q&A is highlighted and the contents of the discussion up to the final draft are explained.

Q24. Are there any precautions to take when telling a minor child about HBOC?

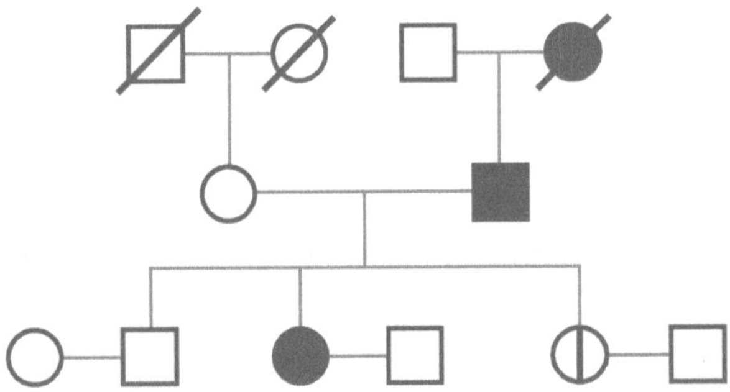

The initial question was "I am concerned about my child," to which the following answer was generated. "After a diagnosis of HBOC, dealing with your child can be an important issue for the family. The first thing that you can do for your child is to familiarize yourself with HBOC. Then, you can consider support for each child that is appropriate to his or her characteristics and your family's situation."

In preparing this answer, the following points were taken into consideration during the drafting stage: (1) "Concerns about children" also vary among individuals and it is necessary to know the background of each client and the intention of the question, (2) it is important for the reader, the "parent," to understand HBOC, because correct knowledge can alleviate concerns and make a satisfactory decision, and (3) the answers were provided in ambiguous terms, assuming that readers in a variety of situations would be able to read them.

During the discussion at the PPI, however, some participants commented that "understanding correctly and how to communicate to the child are two different issues," "isn't the place of genetic counseling to be able to discuss this with the child even if you don't understand it," and "what is being said is not being conveyed. The reason for this divergence in the interpretation of the answers is that "child" can be interpreted in two ways: (1) as a biological or spiritual relationship between a child and a parent, such as a son or a daughter, or (2) as a social relationship, such as a young person. The reason for this is that it is unclear which answer is intended to convey which meaning. Therefore, the question was changed to "Are there any precautions to take when telling a minor child about HBOC?" This was answered as follows:

"When you tell your minor child about HBOC, it is important to consider the child's growth, personality, family, and your own situation, to simulate the situation beforehand, and to be frank without deceit. As an additional note, it is recommended that you do not try to tell the child everything at once, but rather tell them little by little, and that you repeat the explanation while observing the child's understanding and reactions. If your child asks you a question that you are not yet ready to talk about or face, tell them honestly that you are willing to tell them but are not yet ready, for example, "I can't talk about it now, but I will tell you when I am ready. If the child responds with a refusal, such as "I don't want to talk," when you try to tell them, say something like, "Whenever you want to talk, just let me know," and wait until the child changes their mind."

This type of message was devised so that the answers would be specific and close to the concerns of the parties about what they, as parents, should tell their children.

7.4 Commitment to the Guidebook

To ensure that the guidebook reaches a large number of readers, the following points were considered. First, regarding the title, there were various opinions on PPI (e.g., bring the name of the disease to make it easier to understand, Let's know! Is a good active message, whereas "for Patients and Families" does not cover the entire public, the term "guidelines" is too rigid, and based on these opinions), we decided to use "Let's learn about hereditary breast cancer and ovarian cancer! A Guidebook for Everyone." The price of the guideline was set at 1900 yen plus tax to make it affordable to the general public compared with most medical guidelines sold in Japan which cost more than 3000 yen. Furthermore, we were concerned about the size of the guidebook, as existing medical guidelines are B5 in size, which is too large to carry around. In the hope that if the guidebook is carried by patients and the public, the medical community will be prepared to respond, and both parties will carefully read the guidelines to increase their understanding of HBOC. The guidebook was printed in A5 size so it could be carried in a bag, particularly a woman's bag.

7.5 Feedback from the Creation of the Guidebook

The following comments were received from the medical professionals involved in the creation of the guidebook. "It was an opportunity for me to reflect on my explanations in genetic counseling, wondering if I am communicating what I talk about with clients in genetic counseling in an easy-to-understand manner. Because of the diversity of the parties involved, I felt that it is important to provide information that focuses on fundamentally unwavering answers and to help them come up with the answers that seem best to them. Cogent knowledge based on data and evidence is necessary, but it should not be a one-sided and arrogant opinion of the medical staff." Conversely, the following comments were received from the general public and parties involved in preparing the report. "Thank you very much for understanding the position of patients and families taking our opinions and suggestions into consideration, and for allowing us to work together to create this guideline. It also made me aware of the need for many patients and their families to have the correct knowledge and to be positive and tell the medical professionals." These impressions are the most important things we have gained through the creation of this guidebook. We had hoped to create a book that would be truly appreciated by HBOC patients and their families and to be appreciated by those who hold it in their hands. We are convinced that we have fulfilled our aim to create a book that will be truly appreciated by HBOC patients and their families, and one that will be passed on to their friends and employers to be widely read and used by the general public.

Acknowledgments The author would like to express their sincere gratitude to the Health and Labour Sciences Research Grant (Comprehensive Research Project for the Promotion of Cancer Control) "Research on the Development of a Preemptive Medical Care Delivery System for Hereditary Tumors Using Genome Information" group, its representative Prof. Akihiro Sakurai, JOHBOC and President Prof. Seigo Nakamura, and all of the members of the preparation committee, collaborators, and the public for their support in preparing this guidebook.

Chapter 8
2021 Annual report on the BRCA Nationwide Registry Project in the Japanese Organization of Hereditary Breast and Ovarian Cancer (JOHBOC)

Masami Arai and Seigo Nakamura

Abstract To describe the clinical features of hereditary breast and ovarian cancer (HBOC) and *BRCA* pathological variants in Japan, a nationwide registry project was launched by the Japan HBOC Consortium since 2015. From 2019, the main registry project institute was transferred to the Japanese Organization of HBOC (JOHBOC). The registration project has continued till date. Yearly, the registration data, collected until the end of August, are compiled in a dataset. Here, we report the results of the sixth dataset in 2021.

In 2021, 48,038 individuals who underwent BRCA genetic testing and blood relatives who developed cancer from 105 medical institutions in Japan were registered. Of these, 12,976 individuals underwent BRCA genetic testing for the first time in their families. Of these, 16.4% developed pathological variants in *BRCA1/2*, and 3.6% were cases of uncertain pathological significance. Variants of unknown significance (VUS) included inconclusive diagnoses. For insurance coverage in Japan, each diagnostic criterion for conducting BRACAnalysis indicated a positive rate of ≥20%.

Overall, 188 and 430 individuals who underwent risk-reducing mastectomy (RRM) and risk-reducing salpingo-oophorectomy (RRSO) were enrolled, respectively. From 2022, the mutation positivity rate could not be calculated because mutation-negative patients were not registered.

There is a need to report a wider range of information because cases of prostate or pancreatic cancers, which are recently being covered under medical insurance, also has to be registered. Therefore, cooperation is required among clinical depart-

M. Arai (✉)
Department of Clinical Genetics, Juntendo University Graduate School of Medicine, Bunkyō, Japan
e-mail: ms-arai@juntendo.ac.jp

S. Nakamura
Division of Breast Surgical Oncology, Department of Surgery, Showa University School of Medicine, Tokyo, Japan

A. Sakurai et al. (eds.), *Practical Guide to Hereditary Breast and Ovarian Cancer II*, https://doi.org/10.1007/978-981-96-4329-5_8

ments to ensure clinical information input. Furthermore, follow-up registration is not being fully documented because of the extensive time and burden required in the yearly documentation. However, the data will be fundamental and important for use in routine clinical practice.

Keywords BRCA1/2 · HBOC · Database · JOHBOC · Registration

8.1 The Japanese Organization of Hereditary Breast and Ovarian Cancer (JOHBOC) National Registration Project

In Japan, about 4.2% of individuals with breast cancer have *BRCA1* or *BRCA2* mutations [1]. Hereditary breast and ovarian cancer (HBOC) is a syndrome of susceptibility to cancer, mainly breast and ovarian cancers, caused by germline mutations in *BRCA1* or *BRCA2*. It is well known that the frequency of *BRCA1* and *BRCA2* genetic mutations in the general population, pathological variants characteristic of regions, and interactions with lifestyle and environment vary among countries and regions.

In a former Japan Breast Cancer Society group study, Nakamura et al. enrolled 320 patients with a family history of breast cancer from seven centers nationwide, between 2012 and 2013. Among those who underwent *BRCA1/2* genetic testing, 30.7% and 6.2% had pathological variants and variants of unknown significance (VUS) [2]. To further develop and expand this previous study, experts from the Departments of Gynecology and Genetic Medicine as well as Breast Medicine collaborated to establish the Japan HBOC Consortium and initiated a nationwide registry. In October 2013, a registry committee was established in the Japan HBOC Consortium, and a national registry project was initiated. In February 2015, a pilot registry was conducted at four facilities to which members of the registry committee belonged, to validate the registry system. The pilot registry enrolled 965 individuals, 846 families, and their blood relatives who developed cancer, with a total of 3935 participants [3]. Subsequently, the registration system was improved and the first national registry was officially implemented in August 2016. Then, a total of 7188 individuals and their blood relatives were registered in seven centers nationwide, including 1557 families and 1718 individuals. In January 2019, the JOHBOC took over the registry that was previously managed by the Japan HBOC Consortium. JOHBOC, established in August 2016, was to maintain and expand the healthcare delivery system for patients with or suspected of having HBOC and their families. The organization also contributes to the improvement of preventive medicine and healthcare in the nation.

The registry uses a template developed jointly by the JOHBOC and National Clinical Database (NCD). The targeted entry individuals were those who had undergone *BRCA* genetic testing (including mutation-negative individuals) and their second-degree relatives or cousins who had developed any cancers.

Inputs for the individuals include history of cancer, pathological findings of cancer, treatment history, and genetic test results, and for blood relatives, mainly hearsay history of cancer. This multicenter study was conducted after obtaining approval from the ethics committee of each medical institution. The participants provided consent to participate in the study, and their *BRCA1/2* genetic test results and clinical information as well as those of their blood relatives were captured using the template. All entered data were anonymized and transmitted to the NCD of all medical institutions. Registration data for all patients were updated annually. In addition, registered data of patients must have been compiled for each year by the end of August, which is the deadline [4, 5].

8.2 The 2021 National Registration Data Summary

The summary of the national registry data compiled in September 2021 is reported. A total of 48,038 individuals were registered, including 14,157 individuals who underwent BRCA genetic testing from 121 medical institutions nationwide as well as their relatives (Table 8.1). There were 2167 individuals with mutation-positive results including 1062 individuals with *BRCA1* pathological variant-positive results, 1094 with *BRCA2* pathological variant, and 11 with both *BRCA1* and *BRCA2*

Table 8.1 Registered cases in chronological order

	Register for an examination	Nationwide registration					
	2015.2	2016.8 (1st)	2017.8 (2nd)	2018.8 (3rd)	2019.8 (4th)	2020.8 (5th)	2021.8 (6th)
Participating institutions	4	7	35	69	62	93	105
Total registered persons	3935	7118	11,711	16,530 (+4,819)	15,612 (−918)	28,846 (×1.85)	48,038 (×1.67)
Individuals	965	1718	2747	3994 (+1247)	3929 (−65)	7780 (×1.98)	14,157 (×1.82)
Families	846	1557	2433	3586 (+1153)	3629 (+43)	7225 (×1.99)	13,414 (×1.86)
BRCA1 mutation–positive person	135	218	265	429 (+164)	398 (−31)	726 (×1.82)	1062 (×1.46)
BRCA2 mutation–positive persons	119	197	214	319 (+105)	299 (−20)	645 (×2.26)	1094 (×1.70)
Both *BRCA1*+*BRCA2* mutation–positive persons	1	1	3	6	6	7	11 (×1.57)

( ): Change from the previous year

pathological variants. Compared to the previous year, the enrollees increased 1.67 times to 19,192.

8.2.1 *Results of the BRCA Genetic Testing*

Of the 14,157 individuals, 12,976 underwent *BRCA1/2* genetic testing for the first time in their families. Of the 12,976 individuals, 2129 (16.4%) had pathological variants in *BRCA1* or *BRCA2* (Fig. 8.1). *BRCA1*, *BRCA2*, and both *BRCA1* and *BRCA2* occurred in 1044 (8.0%); 1074 (8.3%); and 11 (0.1%) individuals, respectively. In addition, four patients with *BRCA2* pathological variants had two pathological variants. The total mutation-positive rate has been decreasing over the years (19.4% in 2020 registry). This decline can be attributed to two main reasons: (1) more people are undergoing BRCA genetic testing for use as a companion diagnostic, to use poly(ADP-ribose) polymerase (PARP) inhibitor, whereas those not suspected of having HBOC based on clinical information are also undergoing BRACAnalysis and (2) from April 2020, coverage of BRACAnalysis by insurance began, and if clinical criteria are met, the cost of BRCA genetic testing may be less than 100,000 yen (less than approximately 660 USD, as on April 6, 2024). Although the enrollment of mutation-negative individuals may not be as complete as those who tested positive, the mutation-positive rate was examined for each condition that is covered by insurance. The pathogenic variant positivity rate was found to be greater than 20% for all items, which is considered an appropriate criterion for BRACAnalysis (Table 8.2) [6]. Frequent *BRCA1* and *BRCA2* pathological variants (that is, ten or more variants are registered) are listed in Tables 8.3 and 8.4.

VUS was also observed in 462 (3.6%) patients, and its frequency decreased compared to that of the previous year (5.3% in 2020). This decline may be due to the accumulation of data from functional and segregation analyses reports, used to update the assessment results of VUS. The resolution of VUS is an important issue as BRACAnalysis is also used as companion diagnostic.

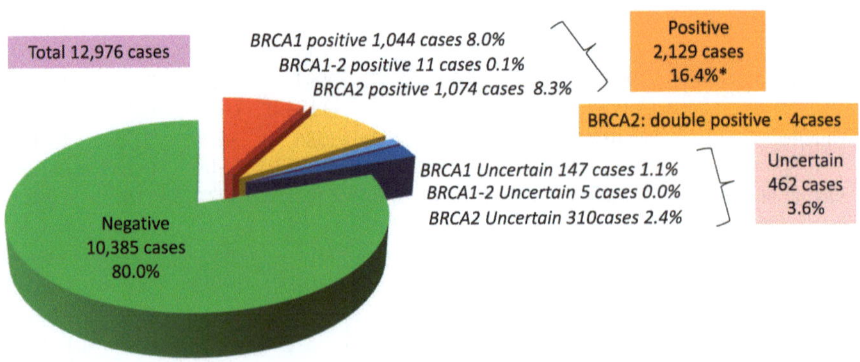

Fig. 8.1 The results of BRCA1/2 genetic test in individuals who were the first to undertake the test in their family

Table 8.2 Mutation rate of each clinical condition for the testing criteria when *BRCA* genetic testing is recommended and public health insurance covers, according to the 2021 JOHBOC registration data

Clients who satisfy one of the following conditions at least one of the following conditions (including duplicates of other conditions)		*BRCA1/2* positive	*BRCA1* positive	*BRCA2* positive	*BRCA1/2* negative	total	Mutation rate (%)
Patients with breast cancer with the following conditions	Onset age <45 years	5	549	580	4541	5675	20.0
	Triple-negative breast cancer, <60 years	0	420	93	1396	1909	26.9
	Double or more primary lesions	2	209	242	1753	2206	20.5
	At least one patient within third-degree relatives with breast or ovarian cancer	9	728	692	4776	6205	23.0
Patients with ovarian, tubal, or peritoneal cancer		3	351	163	1202	1719	30.1
Patients with male breast cancer		0	2	16	70	88	20.5

*Mutation rate in individuals who satisfy at least one of the following conditions

8.2.2 Special Variants

A special variant, *BRCA2,c.658_659del,* registered as pathogenic in Clinvar (ClinVar: Variation ID: 9342), also exists. On the other hand, BRACAnalysis reports this as a "special interpretation," and patients with this variant are not eligible for PARP inhibitors. This is because, according to the Myriad genetic testing report, "though germline carriers of the mutation have a significantly increased risk of breast cancer in comparison with the general population, this risk is not as high as what is typically observed for BRCA2 germline mutation carriers (Myriad internal data)." Therefore, this variant should be classified as pathogenic, not VUS.

Other variants have been registered under different interpretations such as

BRCA1; c.5557 T > A; (p.Tyr1853Asn): deleterious 1; suspected deleterious 2; VUS 1:(n: registration cases in JOHBOC); and conflicting interpreted as ClinVar.

BRCA1; c.2726A > T (p.Asn909Ile); VUS 1; favor polymorphism 1, BRCA1; c.4729 T > C, (p.Ser1577Pro): VUS 1, favor polymorphism 2; were also observed (each number shows the number registered from nationwide institutions in the 2021 version).

Table 8.3 Frequently registered pathogenic variants more than ten times in *BRCA1*

No	Interpretation*	Exon-int. no.	Base change	Amino acid change	2021 Registered	2020 Registered
1	1	5	c.188T>A	p.Leu63*	241	179
2	1	11	c.2800C>T	p.Gln934*	90	67
3	1	11	c.2389_2390del	p.Glu797Thrfs*3	32	25
4	2	24	c.5558A>G	p.Tyr1853Cys	22	18
5	1	11	c.3442del	p.Glu1148Argfs*7	18	10
6	1	3	c.131_132del	p.Cys44*	17	11
7	2	16	c.4964C>T	p.Ser1655Phe	13	8
8	2	19	c.5154G>T	p.Trp1718Cys	13	6
9	1	11	c.2269del	p.Val757Phefs*8	12	6
10	1	20	c.5278-1G>A		12	10
11	1	20	c.5278-1G>C		12	8
12	1	11	c.2075_2076del	p.His692Argfs*19	11	7
13	1	11	c.3640G>T	p.Glu1214*	11	9
14	1	8	c.456_457del	p.Ser153Cysfs*5	10	10
15	1	12	c.4120_4121del	p.Ser1374*	10	7

*; 1: Pathogenic, 2: Likely pathogenic

Table 8.4 Frequently registered pathogenic variants more than ten times in *BRCA2*

No.	Interpretation*	Exon-Int. no.	Base change	Amino acid change	2021 Registered	2020 Registered
1	1	13	c.6952C>T	p.Arg2318*	122	70
2	1	11	c.5576_5579del	p.Ile1859Lysfs*3	100	62
3	1	23	c.9076C>T	p.Gln3026*	66	44
4	1	20	c.8504C>A	p.Ser2835*	50	31
5	1	11	c.5645C>A	p.Ser1882*	42	26
6	1	10	c.1813del	p.Ile605Tyrfs*9	39	24
7	1	23	c.9117G>A	p.Pro3039=	34	19
8	2	18	c.8023A>G	p.Ile2675Val	23	15
9	1	10	c.1278del	p.Asp427Thrfs*3	22	15
10	1	11	c.6405_6409del	p.Asn2135Lysfs*3	21	9
11	1	15	c.7558C>T	p.Arg2520*	21	12
12	1	11	c.2808_2811del	p.Ala938Profs*21	18	13
13	1	11	c.5482_5486del	p.Lys1828Valfs*4	15	9
14	1	25	c.9382C>T	p.Arg3128*	13	7
15	1	3	c.316+2T>C		12	4
16	1	5	c.475+1G>A		11	8
17	1	11	c.5722_5723del	p.Leu1908Argfs*2	11	6
18	1	20	c.8589dup	p.Ala2864Serfs*5	11	11
19	1	20	c.8629G>T	p.Glu2877*	11	8

*; 1: Pathogenic, 2: Likely pathogenic

There are also scattered reports of "inconclusive," with seven registered for *BRCA1* and three for *BRCA2*. Of these, c.(5277 + 1_5278–1)_(*1383_?) is the third most frequently registered (nine times) in VUS for *BRCA1*. The multiplex-ligation-dependent probe amplification (MLPA) method is widely used to analyze large deletions and duplications in exon units, while Myriad uses a unique method known as the binding analysis for the regulation of transcription (BART) method. Regarding the "inconclusive," the results of this fragment analysis shows an atypical pattern, suggesting a large rearrangement; however, the accurate mechanism of unusual results remains inconclusive. The "inconclusive" results, which are currently classified as VUS, showed 7.0% and 10.8% of all VUS in *BRCA1* and *BRCA2*, respectively.

8.2.3 Clinical Background Characteristics of Patients with BRCA1/2 *Mutation-Positive Results*

Of the 12,976 individuals who had undergone initial BRCA genetic testing in their families, 12,647 with known clinical information were compared in terms of gene mutation positivity rates as well as by clinical information, based on the Myriad prevalence table (Table 8.5). The positivity rate was higher in Japanese individuals (Table 8.5, total column) than Westerners, as reported in Myriad prevalence table

Table 8.5 Medical history and BRCA pathogenic variant detection rate among individuals according to the 2021 registration data

Family history	Among 1st – or 2nd-degree relatives				No family history of breast and ovarian cancer	Family history in only 3rd-degree relatives
Breast cancer<50 years	–	+	–	+		
Ovarian cancer at any age	–	–	+	+		
Proband history						
Breast cancer ≥50 years, no ovarian cancer	53/863 6.4%	80/556 14.4%	40/210 19.0%	15/45 33.3%	86/1711 5.0%	10/131 7.6%
Breast cancer <50 years, no ovarian cancer	245/1500 16.3%	337/1141 29.5%	159/338 47.0%	80/138 58.0%	374/3529 10.6%	31/283 11.0%
Ovarian cancer at any age, no breast cancer	36/149 24.2%	41/77 53.2%	100/153 65.4%	17/19 89.4%	147/936 15.7%	5/30 16.7%
Breast cancer and ovarian cancer at any age	44/80 55.0%	23/41 56.1%	34/40 85.0%	12/13 92.3%	54/167 32.3%	4/19 21.1%
Male breast cancer at any age	4/15 26.7%	5/12 41.7%	0/1 0.0%	1/2 50.0%	7/54 13.0%	1/4 25.0%
No breast cancer or ovarian cancer	7/72 9.7%	14/102 13.7%	12/70 17.1%	9/30 30.0%	8/108 7.4%	1/8 12.5%

(The total detection rate was 16.6% [2096/12647])
※Excluding cases in which ages of the onset of breast cancer are unknown

[7]. On the other hand, Japanese women had a 6.4% positivity rate for first-primary breast cancer, even among those aged over 50 years with no family history of HBOC-related cancer (this proportion is reported as 2.2% in Myriad prevalence table) [7].

Among *BRCA* mutation–positive breast cancer cases with clear pathological findings, 69.3% of *BRCA1* mutation-positive cases were triple-negative breast cancer (TNBC) cases. On the other hand, 76.0% of *BRCA2* mutation-positive cases were luminal type.

In breast cancer cases, the contralateral breast cancer incidence rate was 2.6%/year and 1.8%/year in *BRCA1* and *BRCA2* mutation-positive patients, respectively; a six-to-nine-fold risk compared to 0.28%/year in *BRCA* mutation–negative patients (Table 8.6). The risk of developing breast cancer during the follow-up period among never-exposed *BRCA1/2* pathological variant carriers was 6.5% per year, with a mean age at examination of 40.5 years and a mean observation period of 2.2 years (Table 8.7). Further long-term observation is required.

For ovarian cancer, the frequencies of serous adenocarcinoma were 88.8%, 86.0%, and 63.7% for *BRCA1*-positive, *BRCA2*-positive, and *BRCA*-negative cases, respectively, among cases with a known histopathologic type. In terms of advanced stages of ovarian cancer, patients with advanced *BRCA* mutation–positive ovarian cancer tended to have a higher proportion of stages III/IV, with 83.2%, 83.8%, and 76.9% for *BRCA1* pathological variant-positive, *BRCA2* pathological variant-positive, and *BRCA1/2* mutation-negative cases, respectively.

Table 8.6 Incidence of contralateral breast cancer in patients with unilateral breast cancer (female) (2021)

	BRCA1 and *BRCA2* positive	*BRCA1* positive	*BRCA2* positive	*BRCA1/2* negative
Patients with unilateral breast cancer	4 cases	503 cases	613 cases	7150 cases
Patients who developed contralateral breast cancer after genetic testing	1 case	23 cases	20 cases	20 cases
Observation period after genetic testing (average)	0.1~12.1 years	0.0~16.4 years	0.0~16.0 years	0.0~22.2 years
	(4.8)	(1.8)	(1.8)	(1.0)
Incidence (person/person/year)	1/19.2	23/881.6	20/1101.6	20/7197.6
	5.2%/year	2.6%/year	1.8%/year	0.28%/year
Background				
Onset age of patients at the first breast cancer diagnosis (average)	34~78 years	23~84 years	19~80 years	17~88 years
	(53.8 years)	(43.2 years)	(44.4 years)	(47.1 years)
Cases that underwent RRSO (onset of contralateral breast cancer with RRSO)	3 cases (1 case)	107 cases (11 cases)	113 cases (13 cases)	16 cases (0 case)
Excluded cases that underwent RRM	1 case	122 cases	8 cases	cases

Table 8.7 Incidence of breast cancer after genetic testing in unaffected *BRCA1/2* mutation carriers (females) (2021)

Unaffected carriers*	274 cases
Observation period after genetic testing (average)	0–19.5 years (2.2 years)
Age at the time of genetic testing (average)	18–82 years old (40.5 years)
Breast cancer incidence (rate) after testing	40 cases/620 (person/year) (5.6%/year)
Ovarian cancer incidence (%)	4 cases/620 (person/year) (0.6%/year)
Other cancer cases (%)	3 cases/620 (person/year) (0.5%/year)
BRCA1 positive: 33 cases, *BRCA2* positive: 14 cases	
Opportunity of breast cancer detection (including overlapping)	MRI: 15 cases, MMG: 15 cases, palpation: 19 cases, ultrasound: 14 cases, CT: 1 case, MMT: 2 cases, self-detection: 2 cases, puncture biopsy: 2 cases
Breakdown of other cancers	Cecal cancer, uterine cancer, MALT lymphoma

*Excludes cases with unknown observation period and includes previously diagnosed cases

8.2.4 *Risk-Reducing Surgery in Practice*

For risk-reducing mastectomy (RRM), 258 patients were enrolled, and 18 (7.0%) were found to have latent breast cancer in the resected specimen, based on the post-operative pathological examination. In 188 out of the 258 patients (mean age, 44.0 [24–79] years) with known observation period (mean observation period, 25.4 [0–101.8] months), three developed breast cancer postoperatively,. The risk of breast cancer development from the residual mammary gland was 0.8%/year.

For risk-reducing salpingo-oophorectomy (RRSO), 559 patients were enrolled, and 10 (1.8%) developed latent ovarian cancer in the resected specimen (excluding serous tubal intraepithelial carcinoma [STIC]), based on the postoperative pathological examination. Out of the 559 patients, 430 (mean age at surgery, 49.0 [32–78] years) had known observation period (mean observation period, 28.0 [0–184] months). Of the 430, peritoneal cancer developed postoperatively in 1, and the risk of developing peritoneal cancer was 0.1%/year.

8.3 Published Articles Using Registration Data Based on the 2021 or Preceding Versions

Ohsumi et al. reported the actual status of RRM in BRCA pathological variant carriers using 2019 version registration data. Of the 687 pathological variant carriers, 90 (13.1%) had undergone RRM. Multivariate analysis showed that having a pathological variant in *BRCA1*, a history of breast cancer, having children, undergoing contrast-enhanced magnetic resonance imaging (MRI) screening, and undergoing genetic testing were independent factors of undergoing RRM when RRM and BRCA genetic testing were not covered by public medical insurance [8].

Guo and Miki et al. revealed that out of 158 VUSs registered in JOHBOC database (not in ClinVar, an international standard database), seven *BRCA1* variants(p. Gl272Gly, p.Lys1095Glu, p.Val1653Leu, p.Thr1681Pro, p.Phe1761Val, p.Thr1773Ile, and p.Gly1803Ser) and four *BRCA2* variants (p.Trp31Gly, p p.Ser2616Phe, p.Tyr2660Cys, and p.Leu2792Arg) were determined to be pathogenic using conventional homologous recombination assay [9].

Yamazawa et al. performed a clinical study of *BRCA2*, c.7847C > T (p.Ser2616Phe) with additional clinical data from ten individuals from seven families, supported by the JOHBOC registration committee. Moreover, they used the MANO-B method, a functional analysis, to determine that this variant is likely pathogenic [10]. A further segregation study for this variant is currently underway to evaluate the clinical significance of the variant in more detail. Matsumoto et al. reviewed the comparison of clinical factors pre- and post-medical insurance coverage for BRCA genetic testing and RRSO [11].

8.4 Future Perspective

The registration of negative *BRCA* recipients will be terminated after the 2021 version, and only subjects with *BRCA* mutation–positive or VUS will be registered from the next round. Although this revision of the registration strategy is to reduce the burden of the dramatic increase in the number of cases that would be registered, it will no longer be possible to calculate the positivity rate. Providing clarification regarding the results of genetic testing such as VUS, "inconclusive" or "special interpretation" is necessary for better clinical management.

In addition, follow-up data input is inadequate, and prospective chronological follow-up of events is insufficient. Furthermore, as the target population expands, including patients with prostate or pancreatic cancer, the number of relevant medical departments should also increase, as well as collaboration between several staff. We hope for an increase in the number of participating facilities in this registry project and that the database develops to better reflect the actual HBOC clinical practice in Japan.

Acknowledgments We thank the JOHBOC Registration Committee [Committee]: Takayuki Enomoto (Niigata University Graduate School of Medical and Dental Sciences), Tadashi Nomizu (Hoshi General Hospital), Akihiro Sakurai (Sapporo Medical University), Masayuki Sekine (Niigata University Graduate School of Medical and Dental Sciences), Hiroyuki Nomura (Fujita Health University), Megumi Okawa (St. Luke's International Hospital), Hiraku Kumamaru (University of Tokyo), Takeo Kosaka (Keio University), and Masato Ozaka (Cancer Institute Hospital), [Secretariat of JOHBOC]: Eriko Shimamoto (Showa University) and Shiro Yokoyama (Showa University).

We also acknowledge the 121 participating institutions that contributed their data to our 2021 registry: Aichi Cancer Center Hospital, Asahikawa Medical University, Cancer Institute Hospital, Chiba University, Ehime University, Fujisawa City Hospital, Fujita Medical University, Fukui

Prefectural Hospital, Fukui University, Fukushima Medical University, Gifu University, Gunma Prefectural Cancer Center, Hamamatsu Medical Center, Hamamatsu University School of Medicine University Hospital, Hiroshima City Hospital, Hiroshima Prefectural Hospital, Hiroshima University, Hokkaido Cancer Center, Hokkaido University, Hoshi General Hospital, Hyogo Cancer Center, Hyogo Medical University, Hyogo Prefectural Amagasaki General Medical Center, Ibaraki Prefectural Hospital, Ishikawa Prefectural Central Hospital, Iwate Medical University, JA Hiroshima General Hospital, Japan Community Health Care Organization Sagamino Hospital, Japanese Red Cross Aichi Medical Center Nagoya Daini Hospital, Japanese Red Cross Ishinomaki Hospital, Japanese Red Cross Medical Center, Japanese Red Cross Nagoya Daiichi Hospital, Japanese Red Cross Saitama Hospital, Japanese Red Cross Wakayama Medical Center, Japanese Red Cross Yamaguchi Hospital, JCHO Saitama Medical Center, Jisenkai Aizawa Hospital, Juntendo University, Kagawa Prefectural Central Hospital, Kagawa University Hospital, Kagoshima University Hospital, Kanagawa Cancer Center, Kanazawa University, Kansai Medical University, Kansai Rosai Hospital, Kawasaki Medical School, Keio University, Kindai University Hospital, Kitakyushu Municipal Medical Center, Kitano Hospital, Kitazato University, Kochi Medical Center, Kochi University, Kokura Medical Center, Kyoto University, Matsushita Memorial Hospital, Mie University Hospital, Miyagi Cancer Center, Nagasaki University, Nagoya City University, Nagoya University, Nara Medical University, Nara Prefecture General Medical Center, National Center for Global Health and Medicine, National Hospital Organization Kyoto Medical Center, National Hospital Organization Kyushu Medical Center, National Hospital Organization Osaka National Hospital, Nihonkai General Hospital, Niigata City General Hospital, Niigata University, Nippon Medical School, Nippon Medical School Musashi Kosugi Hospital, Ogaki Municipal Hospital, Oikawa Hospital, Okayama University, Okazaki City Hospital, Osaka International Cancer Institute, Osaka Metropolitan University Hospital, Osaka University, Sagara Hospital Breast Center, Saiseikai Hyogoken Hospital, Saitama Cancer Center, Saitama Medical Center, Saitama Medical University International Medical Center, Saku Medical Center, Sapporo Medical University, Seirei Hamamatsu General Hospital, Sekishindo Hospital, Shiga University of Medical Science, Shikoku Cancer Center, Shikoku Medical Center for Children and Adults, Shimonoseki Saiseikai General Hospital, Shinshu University, Shiroyama Hospital, Shizuoka Cancer Center, Shizuoka General Hospital, Shizuoka municipal Hospital, Shonan Memorial Hospital, Showa Medical University Hospital, St. Luke's Hospital, St. Marianna University School of Medicine, Tawara IVF Clinic, The Jikei University, Tohoku University Hospital, Tokushima University Hospital, Tokuyama Central Hospital, Tokyo Medical Center, Tokyo Metropolitan Komagome Hospital, Tokyo Saiseikai Central Hospital, Toranomon Hospital, Tosei General Hospital, Tottori University, Toyama University Hospital, Toyota Memorial Hospital, University of Miyazaki Hospital, University of Tsukuba, Yamagata Prefectural Central Hospital, Yamaguchi Rosai Hospital, Yamaguchi University, Yamanashi Prefectural Central Hospital, Yodogawa Christian Hospital, Yokohama City University.

References

1. Momozawa Y, Iwasaki Y, Parsons MT, Kamatani Y, Takahashi A, et al. Germline pathogenic variants of 11 breast cancer genes in 7,051 Japanese patients and 11,241 controls. Nat Commun. 2018;9(1):4083. PMID: 30287823
2. Nakamura S, Takahashi M, Tozaki M, Nakayama T, Nomizu T, et al. Prevalence and differentiation of hereditary breast and ovarian cancers in Japan. Breast Cancer. 2015;22(5):462–8. PMID: 24249303
3. Arai M, Yokoyama S, Watanabe C, Yoshida R, Kita M, et al. Genetic and clinical characteristics in Japanese hereditary breast and ovarian cancer: First report after establishment of HBOC registration system in Japan. J Hum Genet. 2018;63(4):447–57. PMID: 29176636

4. Arai M. The Registration Committee of the Japanese Organization of Hereditary Breast and Ovarian Cancer (JOHBOC). Hereditary breast and ovarian cancer (HBOC) database in Japan, Molecular mechanism and clinical practice. Singapore: Springer; 2021. p. 243–57.
5. Inuzuka M, Arai M, Nakamura S. Registration data of Japanese organization of hereditary breast and ovarian cancer till. Practical guide to hereditary breast and ovarian cancer. 2020;2023:145–54.
6. Guidebook for diagnosis and treatment of hereditary breast and ovarian cancer syndrome 2017. https://johboc, jp/guidebook2017/toc/2-1index/cq1/ (last accessed March 13, 2024) (in Japanese).
7. Myriad Prevalence Tables. (last accessed April 6, 2024) extension //nhppiemcomgngbg-deffdgkhnkjlgpcdi/data/pdf.js/web/viewer.html?file=https%3A%2F%2Fs3.amazonaws.com%2Fmyriad-library%2Fbrac%2Fbrca-prevalence-tables.pdf
8. Ohsumi S, Nakamura S, Miyata H, Watanabe C, Den H, Arai M. Risk-reducing mastectomy for women with hereditary breast and ovarian cancer (HBOC): analytical results of data from the Japanese Organization of HBOC. Jpn J Clin Oncol. 2022;52(11):1265–9. PMID: 35905458
9. Guo Q, Ji S, Takeuchi K, Urasaki W, Suzuki A, et al. Functional evaluation of BRCA1/2 variants of unknown significance with homologous recombination. J Hum Genet. 2023;68(12):849–57. PMID: 37731132
10. Yamazawa K, Sugano K, Tanakaya K, Inoue S, Murakami H, et al. The pathogenic role of the BRCA2 c.7847C>T (p.Ser2616Phe) variant in breast and ovarian. Cancer Sci. 2023;114(7):2993–3002. PMID: 37067535
11. Matsumoto M, Den H, Miura S, Harada A, Nomura H, Arai M, et al. The impact of public insurance on RRSO for HBOC in Japan: a nationwide data study (under review).

MIX
Papier aus verantwortungsvollen Quellen
Paper from responsible sources
FSC® C105338

If you have any concerns about our products,
you can contact us on
ProductSafety@springernature.com

In case Publisher is established outside the EU,
the EU authorized representative is:
Springer Nature Customer Service Center GmbH
Europaplatz 3, 69115 Heidelberg, Germany

Printed by Libri Plureos GmbH
in Hamburg, Germany